BOO
ZESTFUL AGING IN A
STRESSFUL AGE

MERRILL C. HUBBARD PH.D.

ISBN-13: 978-1542856157
ISBN-10: 1542856159

Library of Congress Cataloging-in-Publication Data:
Hubbard, Merrill C.
    boomers' journey: zestful aging in a stressful age/ by
    Merrill C. Hubbard. Ph.D.
    2nd Ed.
    Includes bibliographical references and reference page.
    Aging process. 2. Psychological aspects. 3. Religious
    aspects. I. Title

CONTENTS

PREFACE

It's the spring of 2015 and I'm asking myself why I started writing *Boomers' Journey* in the first place. Originally, I conceived of a small self-help book that would bring to completion the research and writing on the aging process that I started 40 years ago. I intended to do more research to bring my work up to date while taking into account the changes in society that have occurred since then. I also wanted to write from my current perspective: as a man who had reached 70 and gone through many difficult life challenges. I had planned to keep it short and succinct, and it came in at under 100 pages. Those I shared my work with liked it. The concept was strong, the research illuminating, and the exercises that I had created for each chapter fulfilled the requirements of a self-help book. But I couldn't help but feel that it lacked something.

I found out in the process of revising it that what it lacked was heart—my heart. I discovered a good editor and with her encouragement set out once again to write a book about the second half of life that did not hold back and shared my own personal experiences. If I was going to help the boomer generation navigate new territory, I needed to trust my readers enough to honestly divulge all the issues that I faced throughout the process.

What I couldn't have anticipated was the pain I would go through in revisiting the scenes from my own life. I never dreamed that I would have to stop writing because of the emotions that came up so freely. Nor did I think that I would have to walk away from my keyboard and weep—for myself, my son, my ex-wife, and my family of origin. Weep for lost opportunities and unfortunate decisions, the mere knowledge that can only be gained in hindsight. I thought that five years of therapy was enough to help me move on from the sorrow that has been so much a part of my life. Now I think that sorrow is an inescapable aspect of the human experience, perhaps even more so as we age. Perhaps John Irving is right when he laments in *The Hotel New Hampshire* that "Just when you think you are out of the woods, you find that you're not really out of them at all." As I worked my way through the woods of my own life story, *Boomers' Journey* became a catharsis that I did not expect. And so along with research, psychological interpretation, and political commentary, I have included personal memoirs sprinkled throughout the chapters.

As a student of the writings of Carl Jung, I am inclined to see life divided into two halves, each with its own developmental tasks and challenges. The first half requires taking hold of life, developing and sustaining healthy attachment to our parents as we grow up, forging new adult attachments to significant others and friends, giving birth and nurturing children. It may also include giving back to society, and hopefully, finding meaning in life through love and work. The difficulties and rewards of these tasks are the subjects of thousands of books, articles, and lectures.

The second half of life requires us to let go of much of what we acquired during the first half. As we age, we have to navigate a host of obstacles: releasing our children as they leave home and establish their own lives, losing our parents and all the members of the generation before us, sometimes losing the security of regular income, and even what had formerly constituted our life purpose as retirement becomes inevitable. Adding to these changes, our physical and mental capacities wane, eventually leading to that final transition, death. Not as much has been written about the developmental tasks through this half: the challenges of letting go of life and the pain and sorrow that accompany these losses, but also, the potential for a new sense of freedom, of personal growth and enrichment as our integrity is forged through this fire.

Given the sheer numbers of baby boomers and their influence on the rest of the population, I believe that much more literature is on the horizon. This book differs from many of those previously written. Some focus on the results of long term studies and their implications for "successful aging". Others talk about the connections between aging and spiritual practice. Most of these "aging" books put their emphasis on the period of life following retirement, while I have expanded my scope to include a much broader sense of the "second half." I also want to be honest about both the positive and negative aspects of this time of life, and not sugarcoat the real difficulties that exist. My hope is to give the reader some warning of the dangers ahead, but, more importantly, also present options that can make it an exciting and rewarding journey.

In my thirty-seven years as a Marriage and Family Therapist, it was my privilege to help people of all ages deal with the developmental tasks relevant to their particular stage of life. As I grew older, many of my clients grew old along with me, and we began to face the same life tasks. I saw clients who navigated aging with grace and a sense of new purpose, and those for whom bitterness and regret ruined their final years. There were clients who clung to bad marriages out of terror of being alone, and those who recreated their marriages to suit the needs of the different people they and their spouses had become. I also saw clients who knew when to call it quits and leave marriages whose deficiencies only became more apparent over time. Others were left to pick up the pieces after being surprised by a partner's unanticipated abandonment. Some of my clients reveled in the achievements of their children and grandchildren, while others despaired over children who failed to fulfill their expectations. Many had trouble accepting the fact that their children were adults who had to live with the consequences of their own choices. Instead, they sought to rescue them or punish them, as if they were still toddlers.

In short, I was all too rapidly aging, and so were many of my clients, and we both faced the inherent crises and losses that come with life as it moves beyond its midpoint. That midpoint, incidentally, is not a function of any specific age or life event, but occurs when a person begins to look at the time he or she has *left to live*. Faced with that reality, we begin to evaluate what we've done with our lives up to that point, and consider what we want to do with the time left. I worked with so many people who were depressed and regretful about the lives they had led, the mistakes and missed opportunities, the hurt and pain they had never resolved, and their dread of the future. Some feared the emotional repercussions of the losses to come; some feared for their financial survival. And given that we are all living much longer these days, these are realistic fears. In our current world, there is a much longer stretch of time in which to suffer with regrets and lack of meaning, or to find hope in the possibilities that exist if we are open to them.

Recently, I turned 70. For my parents' generation, reaching 70 seemed a major milestone. You'd have outlived most of your older family members and a good number of your peers. This birthday passed with hardly a notice, except that I decided to retire and put full time effort into this book. Only two years older than the first of the Boomers, I struggle with the same kind of issues and worries, past scars, and future fears. With this in mind, I consider myself a member of the boomer generation.

The challenge for all of us is to choose the lives we want to live through this second half, to find our true selves again (or maybe for the first time). I hope to set out ways this period of life can be both dynamic and deeply rewarding, a time for the expression of untapped potential, creativity and personal growth. We will all face the grief of social and physical losses, but if we face those losses with a stronger sense of purpose, our grief will be less all encompassing, less debilitating to our spirit.

The scope of this book moves from the lofty realms of spirituality down to psychological issues, and further down to some of the practical ones as well.

After the initial chapter, which is an introduction to the aging process and the place of the boomer generation within that process, *Life Out of the Fast Lane* gets us started on the journey with the challenge of accepting our age as something to acknowledge rather than deny. We can find strength as we accept a slower pace and make a new commitment to cooperative efforts. Working together needs to replace our history of competition if we are to age well. *Re-Tired Parenting* explores the changes that occur when our children grow into adulthood, and how we can create new and more meaningful relationships with them. *Transformed or Transplanted* focuses on the opportunities to create a whole new life for ourselves during the period of life I call "later maturity." Rather than transplanting our old beliefs and values into this new stage of life, we can transform ourselves into who we were really meant to be. *Comfort or Challenge* is indeed a challenge to all my readers to create a new paradigm for the aging process rather than looking for the closest rocking chair. *They're Only Memories* focuses on those long forgotten or repressed parts of ourselves that continue to cause us pain and regret. This pivotal chapter is one place in the book where I share more of my own life experience. *Acquiring or Downsizing* is a light-hearted look at all the stuff we have accumulated through the years and what makes it so hard to let our "things" go, even when they are more of a burden than a source of joy. *Love in the Time of Later Maturity*, another pivotal chapter, takes a long look at the state of boomer relationships, both past and present, and asks the question: what is the future of love and marriage? *Who is in Your Circle?* explores the importance of maintaining a social circle throughout the aging process, and learning how to forgive and accept forgiveness when relationships have been damaged or ended. *Religion or Spirituality* presents another challenge to move beyond the tradition of "old time religion" and explore the transcendent within ourselves. Finally, *Finding Meaning: Aging with Integrity* summarizes my thoughts on what I feel is the most important task for the second half of life, namely, finding meaning for what has been as we look forward to what lies ahead.

Each chapter includes an exercise, designed to make you think more deeply about the subject matter covered. Each exercise will challenge you to get in touch with your own thoughts, hopes and dreams for the journey ahead. As a man who has been through the wars, has learned some helpful strategies, and experienced what can get in the way of healthy aging, I invite you to follow me through this guide to the rest of your life. May we all celebrate together as we see that *this moment* is the only moment we have, and live it zestfully.

ACKNOWLEDGMENTS

First and foremost, I dedicate this book to my son Wes, and my life partner, Barbara—without whose love and support this book would not have been possible. Special thanks go to Deborah Lott, for her fine editing, and Monika Mira, for her vision and hard work in putting the book together. My deepest gratitude goes to my friend, Greg Wray, for his inspiration, and beautiful cover design. What a team!

BOOMERS' JOURNEY

To laugh often and much; to win the respect of intelligent people and the affection of children; to earn the appreciation of honest critics and endure the betrayal of false friends; to appreciate beauty; to find the best in others; to leave the world a bit better, whether by a healthy child, a garden patch, or a redeemed social condition; to know even one life has breathed easier because you have lived. This is to have succeeded!

--Ralph Waldo Emerson

AGING AND THE BOOMER GENERATION

Memory teases me, evanescent, transforms me in a breath of time into a bride holding fear and hope inside my white voile wedding dress. I am young and breathless with excitement. . . No. I am old and breathless with fatigue. I know; I know, they say. There are problems with being old. But they do not know. Everyone has been a child. All can understand through muffled memory how childhood was. But none has been old except those who are that now.

--Bert Kruger Smith, *Aging in America*

These poignant words reflect both the mystery and the reality of the aging experience. From the moment of birth, all persons are getting older, yet few can envision themselves as old. The aging process is little understood but much maligned. "Old age," write Sydney Callahan and Drew Christiansen in an article entitled *Ideal Old Age*, "is a painful subject in America. For one thing, aging presents difficult and complex problems, and for another, most unforgivably, there's no future in it."[1] The American people have always seen themselves as youthful, as people with a future. America is a young nation, and for most of its history, the majority of its people have been young. However, this is rapidly changing.

The face of aging in the United States is undergoing dramatic and rapid changes, according to a recent report from the U.S. Census Bureau. The older Americans of today are living longer, are achieving higher levels of education than ever before, have lower rates of disability, and are enjoying higher socioeconomic status. And the baby boomers, who began to turn 65 in 2011, threaten to redefine what it means to be an aging American. Looking into the future, it is projected that people age 65 and over will represent 20% of the total U.S. population by 2030, compared with 12% in 2003. Combine this with increasing life expectancy, which in the year 2000 was just 77 years, and you can readily see the trend of an ever-increasing population of Americans 65 years and older.

As a specific generation, boomers are much different than any generation that has come before or since. The Traditionalists, born between 1900 and 1945, faced two major wars and were raised by parents who had survived the Great Depression. They were hard working people who adhered to the rules and conformed to the demands of society. They had a strong focus on the family, were patriotic and had great respect for authority. Conservative in nature, they believed in dedication and sacrifice, and in deference to their parents, were fiscally prudent savers.

By contrast, baby boomers reacted to the Vietnam War, both soldiers and citizens alike, by becoming anti-war and anti-government. They challenged almost every authority and are responsible for bringing about major social changes. Where their parents were hard working, boomers created the 60-hour work week, demonstrating their attitude of "living for work." Growing up with the "American Dream," they reached new heights of consumerism and are often seen as the "selfish generation." In fact, their attitude of spend now, worry later, has caused many boomers to work, at least part time, into their seventies and eighties, because they haven't saved for retirement. Those who do retire, however, put a great deal of time and effort into community and volunteer activities.

Never has there been a generation who focused as much on personal gratification and growth, often at the expense of their families. With such a focus on self, it is not hard to understand why boomers have the highest divorce rate of any other generation as well as the highest rate of second marriages. On the positive side, they are really the first generation to take care of both aging and disabled parents, and at the same time, often have grown children returning home to live.

Whatever negative things can be said about the boomers, they are an extremely powerful economic and political group. This is truly a transformational generation, bridging the gap between the more conservative and rule oriented traditionalists, being the catalyst for tremendous social and political change, and now developing the skills necessary to be part of the technological revolution. Many

Americans fear the "grey tsunami" that is rapidly approaching as more and more boomers reach retirement age and start to put a burden on the economic and health care systems.

It is obvious that the graying of America is a very significant phenomenon, one that will inevitably bring many changes to the American way of life. As the United States becomes more and more a nation of middle-aged and older people, cultural values may also change. Allan Mayer in a *Newsweek* article entitled The *Graying of America* writes that America's frantic worship of the young is bound to decline. "The shifting demographic balance," he writes, "may well erase the stigma the young in America have attached to age and aging. As the ranks of the middle-aged swell in the next few years—while the number of young people continues to drop—it's even possible that a new ethic could emerge.[2]

It is that potential new ethic that I will address in this book. Although change is as inevitable as life itself, it is not my purpose to focus upon these changes as losses, but rather to create an image of optimal aging that sees the aging process as filled with opportunities for creativity and personal growth throughout. Obviously, for many Americans, physical and social losses are as inexorable as the passing years. But for the rapidly growing population of healthy and vital senior Americans, losses are balanced and offset by creative possibilities and potential gains.

When we think of our own aging in more specific terms, we are likely to focus on what has remained stable over time. In many ways we are today what we have always been in terms of natural talents, personal capabilities and endowments. All of these characteristics, of course, have been filtered through the opportunities and adversities that have occurred throughout our lives. We have grown and changed due to our interactions with others, with the environment, and with the myriad challenges that have confronted us. In this sense, life is a process of constantly refining ourselves. We have traveled the breadth of experience, and these travels have changed us, yet have also reinforced what is unchangeable within us. Wordsworth says it this way:

My heart leaps up as I behold a rainbow in the sky
So it was when I was a child, so it is now that I am grown
So shall it be when I am old--or let me die.

We are what we were, and to some extent what we are yet to become. Think for a moment about the things that have remained constant throughout your life as well as those things that have changed. Objects, beliefs, even people who were once very important, don't matter as much now, while others matter more. We have developed new tastes, modified old ones, developed new ideas, new values. We have gained some knowledge, and maybe even some wisdom, and now it is time to apply that to the challenge of aging.

Using this wisdom requires a starting place, the ability to know when the aging process really begins. We could say that it starts when the body has reached stability in terms of physical growth. Or we could connect it to individual perspective, such as when each of us begins to feel that we are aging. It may well be that aging begins the moment we start to experience time differently. The famous gerontologist, Bernice Neugarten, so eloquently expressed this as "time-left-to-live" rather than "time-since-birth." This is a threshold that we all seem to cross while often remaining unaware of that passage until later. Nevertheless, with it comes a whole new set of expectations and concerns for the time ahead, physically, emotionally and financially. To stretch this thinking a bit further, how about the term *old age*? Do we change our definition of *old* in talking about ourselves as opposed to someone else? No matter how we choose to define it, most of us would agree with Oliver Wendell Holmes that ". . .Old age is always 15 years older than I am."

Thus, in creating a new ethic or paradigm for aging and old age, we must also create a more positive designation for this period of life. I am proposing the use of the term *later maturity* as describing and defining the span of time along the aging continuum that incorporates aging, retirement and old age. Later maturity as a working concept reflects the period of time beginning with the fifties and including old age—in short, the second half of life. And the second half brings with it a major developmental issue to be resolved, the dynamics of which make possible a rich and fulfilling conclusion. So it is that life presents new challenges throughout its entirety, and we can continue to grow and find enrichment at any age.

Bonnie Hammer, the NBC Universal Cable Entertainment Group Chairman, is a leading edge boomer who recently turned 65. In a current editorial for *Fortune* magazine, she boldly states the kind of attitude I want to present in this book. Saying that for the first time in ages, she was completely open about her age, she went on to challenge the women in Hollywood to "rewrite the script on aging." Noting that almost 2 million women will reach the "magical age" of 65 this year she defiantly confronts the stereotype of aging women as being "past our prime and ready to be forgotten" and declares the need for change.

She ends her editorial by writing, "I believe that women everywhere would share the same profound sense of freedom and possibility if they simply ignored the constraints of conventional expectations—including what it means to turn 65. Rather than give in to an outdated perception, we would instead write a new chapter, not only for ourselves but for the younger generations that follow. And our voices—seasoned, capable and wise—would be heard loud and clear."[3]

I believe that ageism profoundly affects both men and women, but in different ways. In the same way that aging women are made irrelevant by their changing appearance, aging men are diminished by what is perceived as a lack of sexual prowess and physical strength. If women are pressured to get a face lift or a tummy tuck, it is demanded that men get Viagra. I can't decide which is worse: getting criticized for sagging breasts or for a shrinking penis.

This is why it is so important to create a new image of aging, based on the positive values and qualities that only those of us in later maturity can bring. It is my hope to "write a new chapter" on what makes people of our age both vital and relevant to the future of coming generations. Just as I am focusing the material in this book on the time of life I call later maturity, I am dedicating it to baby boomers everywhere, who by our sheer numbers alone, will force the rest of the population to recognize our power and influence. So now it's time to look into the issues that give *Boomers' Journey* real depth and meaning.

LIFE OUT OF THE FAST LANE

You are only young once, but you can stay immature indefinitely.

--Ogden Nash

The older I grow the more I distrust the familiar doctrine that age brings wisdom.

--H.L.Mencken

I've been driving since before I was 16 years old and now I'm 71. Several years ago, the highway brought me a real epiphany about life in general and driving in particular. The first seemingly innocuous lesson came at the hands of the Highway Patrol. No sooner had I come off the on-ramp and merged into traffic than a black and white was beside me signaling me to pull over. I hadn't even had time to check my rear-view mirror. I do admit that I was going a little fast, but the freeway was relatively empty and conditions were good. Nevertheless, I found a place to pull over, gave the usual solemn acknowledgement of the officer and took my medicine in silence. The guy had a lot of nerve, I'll tell you that, and he didn't even give me any slack for being a senior.

The second lesson came on my way home from the office one evening. I was in the fast lane doing about 70 miles an hour, thanks to the speeding ticket. I had to slow down because there was someone in front of me going a little slower. As I slowed down, I noticed in my rear view mirror that someone was flashing me with their lights over and over. I raised my arms in a "what can I do" motion, not thinking the guy behind could even see me anyway. Well, I looked back and, lo and behold, he is giving me the double finger! That's right, he's flipping me off with both hands. I couldn't believe it. So what did I do? I pulled over before he could ram me from behind. I know crazy behavior when I see it, and I wasn't about to give this guy a chance to do anything irrational (as if the double bird is rational). I used to get angry about people who drive recklessly, or who come up behind me way too fast, but my girlfriend has been on my case for that lately, so I'm trying to get better. I just pulled over and let him be someone else's problem. And you know what? I felt a lot better. I wasn't angry; I was relieved.

Well, what lesson could I have learned from an officer of the law and a lawless cowboy? The lesson is so simple, yet so hard for many of us who continue to do everything the way we used to, because we feel special and entitled in some way. It has finally sunk in that it's time for me to get out of the fast lane and let the younger generation go by. My reflexes aren't that good anymore and my reaction time is a little slower, so it's time to get out of the passing lane, reduce my speed, and enjoy life at a slightly slower pace. Driving in that lane is liable to get me into more trouble, be it a ticket, trouble with someone who wants to go just a little bit faster or feels just a little more important. I've moved over to the next lane and I'm starting to enjoy it.

From a more global perspective, I suggest that it's time for all of us in later maturity to move over and let the younger generation take the places that we once occupied. This doesn't mean that we can't go back there occasionally, or be the leader of the pack now and again. Nor does it mean acting older than we are either. But accepting our age, finding a more comfortable speed at which to travel the rest of our lives, brings more enjoyment and less stress. And we can all do with less stress, right? I know that there are some exceptional people who drive a car, or a company, or other creative endeavors at high speed well into their eighties. But, I'm talking about a way of life that is more suited for the vast majority of people in later maturity, people who have worked hard and raised their children, who now want to read the paper in the morning and wear their slippers just a little longer before pulling out into traffic again. This isn't a matter of giving up and seeing ourselves as too old to do certain things. It is surrendering to the truth that aging is a process that we all go through—some more rapidly than others and with more debilitating consequences—a process that changes our bodies and our minds in ways that turn the early sprint of life into a long-distance race that requires the wisdom and insight to pace ourselves properly.

A case in point for moving over to let others take our place in life is illuminated in the sensational career of guitarist Tommy Tedesco. He was the key figure in the legendary group of studio and session musicians, nicknamed the *wrecking crew*, that played anonymously on innumerable recordings in Los Angeles during the 1960s—everything from Frank Sinatra to the Beach Boys. Described by *Guitar Player* as the most recorded guitarist in history, he played on thousands of records as well as movie and TV soundtracks (you might remember his blazing guitar solo on the theme for Bonanza). In 1992, Tedesco had a stroke that left him partially paralyzed and effectively ended his career as a guitarist. His son, Denny, reported in the 2008 documentary film called *The Wrecking Crew*, that his father told him shortly before his death that the stroke "came at the right time," for he knew it was his turn to step aside and let younger musicians take "his seat" just as he had taken someone else's seat 40 years earlier. This highlights the kind of grace and dignity that comes with accepting the passage of time and knowing when it is our time to step aside for the next generation. Finding new purpose for his life, the following year Tommy Tedesco wrote and published his autobiography, *Confessions of a Guitar Player*. He died in 1997 of lung cancer.

But for those who were born at the end of the post war baby boom, and who are just starting their 50s, it's too early to think about a lateral move into a slower pace of life. Moving over and letting the younger generation take your place in the cultural hierarchy of America may seem like an offensive idea to some, and downright blasphemous to others.

The recent literature on the four generations of American workers indicates that there are some important differences between the Boomers, Generation X and the generation referred to as Millenials. To be specific, there are tensions between these generations that come out in the workplace. Like a smooth hand-off in a relay race, in a perfect world, younger boomers would pass the baton knowing that the next generation would build upon their accomplishments and move toward a goal that will benefit the whole. However, this does not seem to be happening. Younger boomers, much like their older counterparts, seem to be as suspicious of generation xers and millenials as we all were of anyone who was ten years older than us. Nowhere is this more apparent than in the areas of basic work attitudes and technology.

Boomers feel that their experience and knowledge is not respected while xers and millenials feel that their ideas are not given enough attention. Older workers are committed to being at work at acceptable hours, whereas younger workers like to work at their own schedule and at home when possible. Younger co-workers feel that their older colleagues are too slow to embrace technology, and boomers see their younger colleagues as being so focused on technology that it becomes a constant distraction, and doesn't increase their efficiency or productivity. Each generation wants to feel that their different strengths are being acknowledged and utilized but they aren't as willing to work together to create a transfer of knowledge from older to younger workers. As a result, there are growing stereotypes and misperceptions of each generation.

In a recent article on *LinkedIn Pulse*, Chris Morrow, senior consultant for *Peoplebank*, listed the top five unspoken objections that companies have when considering hiring boomers:

1. They are tech-averse.

2. They won't get along with younger members of the team.

3. They are stuck in their ways.

4. They are too expensive and unwilling to accept lower salary requirements.

5. They are too negative.

Extrapolating from my own experience and research, I would infer that these criticisms apply to many other areas of intergenerational conflict. Not all boomers demonstrate these qualities (the youngest boomers are 51), but more than enough to create the stereotype. The metaphor of moving out of the fast lane may translate into accepting that our generation, in its entirety, did not grow up using technology, and therefore we are less adept than younger generations. Middle-aged boomers often feel disrespected and pushed aside by generations that will eventually displace them in the workplace, and take their places in leadership roles in the community and in the family. In my opinion, what looks like animosity is actually the fear of being replaced so easily. This fear creates negativity toward younger generations and prevents the kind of open communication and sharing that is needed. Boomers can seem very entitled and aloof when seen through the eyes of younger peers.

The growing up experiences of generation xers and millenials were much different from those of boomers. Where we faced war and social upheaval, they witnessed a period of family and financial insecurity. Often growing up with a single parent or both parents working, they saw massive lay-offs and corporate downsizing affect their parents. They are the children of MTV and the horror of HIV-AIDS. Millenials (also known as Cyberkids) were conditioned by very involved parents, computers and tremendous technological advances. They are very comfortable and skilled with the ever-changing world of technology, much to the dismay of many boomers. Whereas they can do anything on their phones, we struggle to read the texts that we periodically get. Some of us won't even venture into the world of smartphones unless it is a necessity. This contributes to the feelings that we are just too stuck in our ways. I do have a smartphone, but I constantly wish I was smart enough to use it effectively. Further, I generally try to find my own way before I even think of using the same GPS that my younger friends use to punch in coordinates like they were on the deck of the Starship Enterprise.

Just as I encouraged older boomers to accept their age and move over to provide room for following generations, I am encouraging younger boomers to accept their limitations and be leaders in creating intergenerational communication and understanding. To remain aloof and closed off from younger generations only gives fuel to ageism. Don't be a walking anachronism. Don't be so stuck in your ways that you can't demonstrate your expertise in conflict resolution. Don't be so jaded and negative that you turn off the creative flow essential to the workplace. Maybe you feel as though you've seen it all before, but just maybe it will turn out differently this time. Share the wisdom of your experience, but be open to the ideas and creativity of fresh minds. Be wise enough to see that the future is theirs and our part can be in helping them learn to temper their results-focused brilliance with social responsibility. There is the time and space needed for all three generations to work and play side by side in an atmosphere of mutual respect. I think it needs to start with us.

In a recent interview with 56-year-old astrophysicist Neil deGrasse Tyson, the question was asked, are you afraid of getting older? His response was, "No. I used to dance, but I've had my time as an athlete. This is a different chapter of my life that would have been impossible in my physical prime, but my mental prime is still being developed. I look forward to all that I can contribute to this world because of my age and life experience in a way that would have been impossible at half my age."[1]

Along with moving out of the fast lane and providing leadership for younger generations, those of us in later maturity could greatly benefit from no longer framing every situation as a matter of winning or losing, and in so doing bring a new sense of resolution to the competition that separates us, and eventually defeats us. Competition, of course, is as American as apple pie, in fact it is the *sine qua non* of capitalism. I have no illusions about its importance in a free economy, nor am I suggesting that it is inherently evil. The problem derives from the human reaction to competition: the endless striving to be better than, to have more of, to be more successful than the next person, or for that matter, any person.

One person who has taken a much stronger stand on the dangers of competition is Alfie Kohn, in his book, *No Contest: The Case Against Competition.* Kohn confronts the notion that competition is appropriate, required, and unavoidable in American society, and feels that this has been drummed into us from pre-school to college. He suggests that this view is based on the following four myths:

1. Competition is an unavoidable fact of life.

2. Competition motivates us to do our best.

3. Contests provide the best, if not the only way to have a good time.

4. Competition builds character and self-confidence.[2]

After reviewing over four hundred studies focusing on competition and cooperation, he concludes that "Competition drags us down, devastates us psychologically, poisons our relationships, interferes with our performance. But acknowledging these things would be painful and might force us to make radical changes in our lives, so instead we create and accept rationalizations for competition: It's part of 'human nature.' It's more productive. It builds character."[3] Further, there is no evidence to support the idea that competition is unavoidable for human beings. In fact, the prevailing evidence is that competitive striving increases human isolation, hostility and anxiety, and inhibits personal security, while cooperation teaches people the value of relationships, of working with others toward a mutual goal.

It seems that equating success with victory has become an American ethos. In contemporary business and politics, the idea of winning at all costs has led to all kinds of unethical, illegal and inappropriate behaviors. Just listen to the news at night or surf the internet and you'll see exactly what I mean. Professional sports, our much-watched national form of entertainment, has been the source of numerous allegations and proven instances of cheating and drugging that goes on in the name of "getting an edge." Don't get me wrong, I love to watch sports at both the college and professional level, but sometimes the competition goes a little too far.

As a marriage therapist, I have witnessed how the competition over who earns the most, who does the most around the house, who is right and who is wrong, and sadly, who loves more, can take the joy out of a relationship and lead to endless arguments.

It used to be that this kind of competitiveness was the domain of men, but Kohn questions whether women have truly been liberated through the imitation of men, and the adoption of male values. He boldly states, "For women to pump up their biceps or break into the club of hard-driving money grubbers on Wall Street is a peculiar and sad kind of liberation. For the feminine voice to slide down into a baritone that rasps about being number one is a poor excuse for deliverance."[4]

To relate this to our everyday lives, I am suggesting that the aging process provides the opportunity to put limits on mindless competition and start supporting one another. This would mean moving beyond the egocentric focus of competition and facilitating growth and development from both sides. It would support synergism, the cooperative action of two to achieve an effect of which each is individually incapable. It would mean learning that if you win, I don't necessarily lose, and that another's victory only means that ours is possible as well. It would mean setting firm limits on the senseless cupidity and manic drive to acquire more and more things, and start focusing on personal values. It would mean setting personal integrity and human well-being above winning and losing, above self-aggrandizement. Perhaps if we could all commit to these things, then we could truly commit to each other in a way that brings more joy and fulfillment to everyone.

I believe these to be two of the most important tasks of later maturity: moving out of the fast lane to let the younger generation take its place in the world, and learning how to find peace and joy in loving cooperation and synergy.

EXERCISE #1

STARTING A DAILY JOURNAL

A journal is just a place to keep a written record of your feelings, thoughts, and experiences. If you feel intimidated by the idea of a journal, just begin with it as a diary, describing your day, and soon it will expand beyond that written record into a source of inner wisdom and inspiration. Sometimes you don't know what you really think about a situation until you compel yourself to put it into words. Over the years, I have consistently challenged my clients to start journaling on a daily basis. Write freely and without judgment; the pages will magically come to life with material from your subconscious that you may not have been aware of before. Ken Wilbur, one of the most significant contemporary philosophers and writers in the field of personal growth, states, "Meaning is found, not in outward actions or possessions, but in the inner radiant currents of your own being, and in the release and relationship of these currents to the world, to friends, to humanity at large, and to infinity itself."[1]

As you work through this book, I am challenging you to start your own personal journal, opening yourself to your inner world, and allowing those "radiant currents" to find expression through your writing. To get started, simply open to an empty page, set your pen on the paper and begin to write. This is your journal, so you can write anything you want, about anything you want, and in whatever style you want. As there is no right or wrong to journaling, you are free to create whatever you wish.

Many people, however, feel intimidated by a blank piece of paper and nothing specific to write about. If you need structure, and the whiteness of the paper seems to be engulfing your thoughts and feelings, I will list some prompts to get you started. Think of the paper as a pristine snow field, and you have the perfect snow shoes with which to leave your tracks for the very first time. This is your journey through the second half of life and no one else will leave the same impression in life as you will.

Here are some ideas to launch your journey:

1. List (without censoring or judging yourself) your negative images of aging.

2. List (without censoring or judging yourself) your positive images of aging.

3. Now think back. Where do these images come from and what person do you associate with each?

4. What frightens you about your own aging?

5. What experiences and insights could you be missing by maintaining your perceptions about the aging process?

6. What keeps you from accepting the changes that are occurring as you navigate this stage of life?

7. What resistance are you aware of as you think about the chapter you just read?

8. Are there secrets and regrets that you are carrying into this second half of life?

9. What help do you need to make this a less stressed and more peaceful journey?

Continue to be aware of memories, thoughts and feelings, and let this be the source of your journaling. Many people find it helpful to write first thing in the morning or even to keep a little notepad in their purse or pocket so they can jot down feelings and observations throughout the day. Write about your dreams, write letters to people from your past, write poems, but just let yourself write.

RE-TIRED PARENTING

Your children are not your children.
They are the sons and daughters of Life's longing for
itself.
They come through you but not from you,
And though they are with you yet they belong not to you.
                    --Kahlil Gibran, *The Prophet*

Many of us in later maturity complain about our children, saying that they don't seem to appreciate us, or that they are selfish and don't give us the respect or attention that we gave our parents. Many of us have taken care of elderly and/or dying parents, even though those parents may have been abusive to us in our

47

childhood years, and are deeply hurt that our own children, although raised with love and respect, do not show us the same kind of deference. Some of us are disappointed in the paths that our children have chosen, feeling that they could have done so much better, or, on the other hand, that they are working so much that our grandchildren are suffering. Those who are still working, find it difficult to make time for grandchildren and wonder why our adult children don't make them more available to us, don't bring them over enough, and in general do not seek us out in the way we sought our parents. On the other side are those of us who feel we are being used as a free babysitting service.

If you are in any way like me, you spend a lot of your time worrying about your grown child, wondering if you did as much for that child as you could, and regret the ways you could have been a better parent. You may even wake up in the middle of the night, as I do, remembering something you said or you failed to do in raising your child that might now be causing them emotional pain.

For those who experience these feelings, the words of Gibran can be both corrective and liberating. We cannot make our adult children think as we do, no matter how hard we try. Their generation is so very different from ours, especially with the instant access to information and the ever changing technology that often separates us at the level of respect and understanding. We cannot make them be like us, even if they wanted to be, for their experience of growing up with us as their parents has been, hopefully, very different from our experience. Perhaps it would be great if we had the children of our dreams, but I think it would be much better if we accepted and loved the children that we have. If we can do this we may be able to change our role with our adult children and declare ourselves "parents emeritus" as Elwood N. Chapman writes in his book, *Comfort Zones*. "Declare your own emeritus status openly," he continues, "so that all members will know! To back it up, start refusing 'old-time' responsibilities. Continue to love and enjoy adult children and grandchildren, be available for consultation, but back away from stepping in or bailing out. Like a professor moving away from teaching responsibilities, move away from parenting in the old sense."[1]

To illustrate the possibility of moving away from an outdated parenting style and moving toward becoming a parent "emeritus," I would like you to consider an example from my years of working with clients who found parenting difficult and sometimes painful.

Laura was a woman that I had the privilege of working with for many years. She initially came for treatment after several hospitalizations due to her severe mood swings and early childhood trauma.

We spent the early years of therapy working on past issues, stabilizing her mood swings, and learning how to regulate her sometimes overpowering emotions. She might be laughing at one moment in our session and then suddenly break out in tears or become filled with rage. It was always an adventure to be working with Laura and I was constantly being challenged as a therapist to know when to be supportive, when to offer interpretations, and when to be more directive. Did I mention that she was very intelligent as well? I think I learned as much from her about maintaining a therapeutic alliance than with any other client. Our work together was often painful, many times confusing, but always rewarding in hindsight, and spanned nearly fifteen years.

As we came closer to the end of therapy, the issues became less about her past, and more about current relationships, specifically with her adult son James. Laura would often sob as she talked about the difficulties of her relationship with James, how she felt he was angry and disrespectful of her, and sometimes she doubted whether he loved her at all. He would take a long time to answer her messages and criticize her for being too emotional and clingy if she complained or said that these slights hurt her feelings. She felt he was always criticizing her behavior and pulling away from her or openly annoyed with her for things she said or did. All of her attention was focused on what her son was doing and saying, and the pain and sorrow she experienced in their interactions. Even the comforting and supportive comments from her husband did not seem to give her any relief. She was unable to see things from his point of view and let go of the dream of the kind of relationship she wanted, so that she could focus on the relationship that they had.

She reported that when her son would not recognize Mother's Day or her birthday in the way she wanted, he was saying to her that she was not a good mother and that she was "too much" to cope with. Both of these were her own core beliefs which she projected onto James as if he were making her feel this way. I reminded her on several occasions that these were her issues—issues that we had worked on many times before—and she needed to continue to take ownership, remove the projections, and start accepting her son for who he was, not who she wanted him to be. I presented this to her as letting her son "off the hook" in regards to the way he wanted to respond to her on these special days.

In our work together it became important to look at the nature of her co-dependence with her son, and how all her efforts were in pursuing more contact or greater intimacy or approval from him, only to feel his distance and criticism. She would try again and again to get him to understand her point of view, only to feel that he didn't really care. She would go to elaborate measures to try and please him only to feel that she was unappreciated. Laura was stuck in the pursuer-distancer dynamic, one of the most common, yet challenging patterns in all human relationships, whether it is between husband and wife or parent and child. In this pattern, one person is always trying to get something from another; some kind of need fulfillment, validation or recognition, while the other person reacts with various distancing devices such as procrastinating, forgetting or being avoidant. This dynamic often leaves both sides feeling hurt and angry, and can continue for years or even decades, if it is not dealt with in a manner in which both parties can grow and change the ways they keep the dynamic going.

Fortunately, Laura began to understand these concepts and made some significant changes in the way she interacted with James, which I've listed and explained below. As a result, she no longer feels unloved and unappreciated, and is enjoying a much more satisfying relationship with him, her daughter-in-law, and her grandchildren.

I spoke to her recently and she acknowledged that although things still need a lot of work, she experiences the following:

1. She is not pursuing as much and as a result has been welcomed into her son and his

family's lives on a regular basis. In fact, her son recently said, "I love you being here as part of the family."

2. She stays with her grandchildren one day every week and this has given her a new sense of life purpose. Many times in therapy she felt depressed because of a lack of purpose.

3. She is affirming herself more and has been getting unsolicited affirmations, especially from her daughter-in-law.

4. She is more careful in the way she approaches her son, trying not to ask silly questions which in the past led to irritable responses. She is accepting him for who he is now, and that acceptance is coming back to her.

5. She has more of a life now and so does not feel as needy as before.

6. She is learning how to be grateful for what she has, one of the qualities necessary to be happy in life.

Laura is moving away from her past style of parenting and is opening up to new opportunities. By letting go of all the time and effort she put into pursuing her son, lamenting his distance, and trying to induce guilt for rejecting her, she has more time and energy to create a life for herself. By taking the focus off that one perceived failure, she can develop other aspects of her life. She is beginning to let go of the strong parental attachment to James, and in so doing has created a new sense of purpose in grand-parenting. She is moving away from her over-involvement with her son and allowing him the space to invite her into a new relationship, based on equality and mutual respect. By affirming herself as a caring person and a good mother, she finds that she doesn't need compliments and verbal acknowledgment to come from her son, and this provides the emotional space for these endearments to come from him spontaneously. And finally, her relationship with her husband has been strengthened as she re-directs her attention from being a mother to being a wife and partner, and as they work together in their new role as grand-parents.

In a follow-up conversation with Laura, she emphasized that a starting place in making these changes was when her son indicated to her that he and his wife had purchased a bigger house so that she could live with them. This would have been a dream come true for her in the past, but after careful consideration, she began to realize: "I don't want to live with James." With this declaration, she found the strength she needed to let go emotionally and focus on her own life.

I am not suggesting that every parent and adult child relationship change in the manner that Laura's has. Many of our relationships with adult children continue to be filled with conflict and animosity. Some have been torn apart by addictions and emotional problems that isolate one or both sides. Others remain distant and hostile because of past hurts and injuries, including abuse, that have never been resolved. What I am saying is that the principles listed above can be used to work toward change. If there are more serious problems, the help of a professional may be required.

But for the boomers with the "every day" frustrations and concerns about our changing role as mature parents, I am suggesting that we consider retired parenting as moving away from the burden of worrying or feeling guilty about our adult children. Many of us, like Laura, want to change our old style of parenting and create more of a peer relationship with our kids. We wish to release our children to become the adults they were meant to become; with our help and support, but without the control and over-involvement that many senior parents exhibit. This means finding our own unique life style in the later years, one that is supportive of our children but allows us the freedom to enjoy these years in the way we want.

In the last part of his statements on children, Kahlil Gibran compares parents to bows from which, *"your children as living arrows are sent forth."*[2] The message is clear: we are to release our children to go on their own paths, to fulfill their own destinies.

EXERCISE #2

Changing our relationship with our grown children can be a difficult and sometimes painful process. I would like to suggest writing a letter to your adult child or children that includes the following:

1. Stating what you do and don't like about the relationship.

2. Confessing the resentments you have held and then committing to letting these resentments go.

3. Stating the ways in which you have been hurt in the past and then forgiving completely.

4. Committing to being both a better listener and a better communicator.

5. Asking for forgiveness and forgiving yourself for mistakes you have made in the past.

6. Stating how you would like the relationship to be and then letting go of any attachment to the outcome.

7. Finally, expressing in words that you are releasing them completely to be the person or persons they want to be, and that you will accept them for who they are.

Say good bye and sign your name at the bottom. Do not send the letter; it is meant to be a way of expressing and therefore creating the relationship you wish to have with your child or children. It is meant for you.

TRANSFORMED OR TRANSPLANTED

Age is an issue of mind over matter. If you don't mind, it doesn't matter.

--Mark Twain

In a man's middle years, there is scarcely a part of the body he would hesitate to turn over to the proper authorities.
--E.B. White

As time takes its toll on our bodies and we experience a decrease in physical vigor, attractiveness and abilities, feelings of failure or inadequacy may creep into our awareness. We look in the mirror and wonder if we are aging like fine wine or bad cheese. "What happened to my face?" an ex-girlfriend used to mutter. "It's two inches lower than it used to be." I look down at my stomach and see rolling hills where once there were only flatlands. I know that AARP is promoting the theme that you don't stop growing because you are older, but I didn't think that I was going to grow so much in all the wrong places.

What can we do to stop the physical landslide that is aging? Many of my friends complain that they can no longer work the number of hours to which they were accustomed, that they get tired during the day and can't get as much done as they used to only a few short years ago. Our bodies are not as young as they used to be, and our minds are often unable to cope with these physical changes, our expectations not aging along with our bodies. Dr. Robert Klapper, ESPN Radio Host, has a Saturday program called *Weekend Warrior* that's dedicated to the men and women who can't accept their physical limitations and now are suffering with some form of injury. Many of us demand the same things of ourselves as if we were much younger, but our bodies just won't cooperate. Others seem to fixate on their appearance or a sense of prowess that has long passed, becoming a caricature of the person they once were.

So what are we to do? Some choose to contact the best plastic surgeon in the area or pay the local gym's most aggressive trainer to whip them back into shape. I'd be willing to explore both of these if I could only remember where I left my glasses.

In a world that demands that we become the "best that we can be," a world where sixty is the new forty, and sleeping is a waste of time, later maturity can really be a drag. We don't need to change our diets, or our partners or our wardrobes as much as we need to change significantly our standards of self-evaluation. This may sound absurd, but I am suggesting that we start valuing wisdom over physical powers or beauty. Whatever wisdom we might have gained through the passage of time, must now become the major resource for determining both how we feel about ourselves and how we solve life's problems. The time has come to think things through rather than grabbing our trusty tool belt and getting busy. Studies show that the most successful travelers through later maturity are those who have chosen to change their value hierarchy, now placing the use of their "heads" above the use of their "hands." Though our brains may not work as quickly as they did when we were 25, gains have been made in powers of judgment and discernment. We're less likely to act on impulse or to deny our experience, thinking "this time will be different just because I want it to be." This is the wisdom of facing the present armed with experience, having learned to work and to play smarter. It is the ability to perceive the larger picture, especially in the way we see ourselves and our place in the world.

Does valuing wisdom more than physical strength or attractiveness mean that this stage of life is a time to pull into ourselves and wait to be replaced like the worn out old part I had replaced on my washing machine today? It certainly does not. I was thinking just this morning that I had to try and pull out my washer and take it apart myself, because that is what a man is supposed to do. In fact, my dad made me help him do hundreds of projects just like this. But the reality today is that I am tired and have many other tasks of equal importance to do. I chose to hire a professional. And as I watched the mechanic diagnose the problem, disassemble the outer shell and pull the motor out, replace the broken parts and put the machine back together again, I was sure of two things: One, I could not have done in eight hours what he did in less than an hour. Two, it was the best $140 I had spent in months. He's gone now and I'm back to writing, very happy to have used my head rather than my hands.

What I mean by transformation is an entirely new way of viewing our lives, not just transplanting our old beliefs and values into a slightly older version of ourselves. Five years ago, faced with the same situation, I would have struggled and sweated in trying to do it myself, and used every expletive known to man in the process. Then I would have called the mechanic anyway, out of anger and frustration, and still paid him the $140. Now I realize that I don't have the energy or expertise to get the job done, so rather than fighting the inevitable, I chose to make a simple call.

Mine was a simple change of attitude, a slight value shift that made my life easier. A more complex example of transformation can be found in the tenets and practices of the organization called Alcoholics Anonymous. This self-help group has been responsible for the dramatic change of millions of lives—those caught in the downward spiral of addiction and substance abuse. Though it does not subscribe to any specific moral code or religious affiliation, AA is a deeply spiritual organization that tries to guide it members through the 12 steps; a set of "suggestions" that help its followers move from egotism to humility, self-pity to honesty and personal responsibility, and from intolerance to service to others. I have worked with many of their adherents who demonstrated a complete change of personality as they recognized and confronted their denial, surrendered to their "higher power," and then began to work the steps. Those who are successful in the program recover from a highly destructive disease, regain their health and self-respect, and live productive lives. AA has guided millions of followers through a complete transformation of beliefs, attitudes, and behavior. As a modality for helping people, it also engendered the group therapy movement in America. Further, AA has brought about the metamorphosis of an entire culture's way of thinking about alcohol and drugs.

This organization represents a more global transformation that started with one man—its founder Bill W—and expanded out to the local community and then an entire country. It illustrates my belief that our attitudes and behaviors affect those with whom we associate: family, friends, and the world around us, in a more significant way than we realize. We can give our lives meaning when we welcome the change in values that can make later maturity a time of novelty and creativity.

Transformation that we undertake willingly is one thing, but many people in their later years are forced to make changes that they do not choose and do not necessarily see as positive. They may have to move out of their homes and their neighborhoods for financial or health-related reasons. They are uprooted and literally transplanted into smaller apartments, assisted living facilities, or forced to live with their adult children. When this happens, they have to give up social networks and surroundings with which they have been comfortable, as well as the status they had as younger people. Many must say good bye to long-time friends and others must even leave pets behind. This can be experienced as a devastating loss or part of the inevitable changes that occur throughout the aging process. We all need to cope with the discontinuities that come with getting older, such as moving out of our homes or out of our neighborhoods. But we also have the choice to shift our values in such a way that these changes don't lead us to foster regret and bitterness. There is nothing more painful to watch than a bitter old person whose anger and negativity has pushed everyone, including family, away. Instead, we can embrace these changes as opportunities to transform ourselves from being an aging person into a person of value. We can choose to let go of the feelings of being displaced or brushed aside by the younger generation and become an example for subsequent generations: a teacher, a mentor, someone to guide their way. We can age in a totally different way than our ancestors did; using our experience, our decision-making abilities, and our wisdom to remain vitally involved in our families, our communities, and the world in which we live.

Here are some examples of ways in which every boomer can stay active and involved:

1. Senior Corps is an organization that connects people 55+ with other people and organizations that need their skills and expertise.

2. If you like to build things, try Habitat for Humanity.

3. If you are feeling rejected by the younger generation look into becoming a Foster Grandparent or a Big Brother or Sister.

4. Participate in Meals on Wheels to help in your community.

5. Road Scholars and Global Volunteers are for the more adventurous boomers.

6. Humane Societies and Animal Shelters always need volunteers.

7. Political campaigns, Medical Reserve Corps, and USO Volunteers are for those with specific backgrounds and skills.

We are not yet obsolete. In fact, as boomers, it has been our calling and our mantra to confront established ways of thinking. In this regard, it is up to us to challenge the stereotypes of ageism and present a model of aging that is involved rather than withdrawn, positive rather than negative, and one that finds deep meaning in this stage of life.

This requires that we value ourselves enough not to be put off by rejection. When others don't value our expertise, we must take this as a challenge to continue learning and evolving and becoming more of the persons that we always wanted to be.

Transformation can take many forms. A caterpillar is transformed into a butterfly by a process of nature. Solids can be transformed into liquids with heat as a catalyst, and then again into gases with additional heat. Human beings seem to require an external stimulus, such as a life-changing event or increasing stress to initiate the process of self-transformation. One personal example is a very good friend of mine whom I met about ten years ago, after she had moved from Long Island, New York, to Southern California.

Babs is a very strong, leading edge boomer woman, divorced and living independently. At that time, she was residing in a beautiful home situated on a golf course on Long Island. Her children were grown and living on their own, and she had a wonderful group of friends with whom she planned on taking future cruises. In fact, the group had already cruised to Mexico and Europe, returning with many fond memories of great times together.

Even the vacation in which she fell and broke her arm did not prevent her from having a good time and recounting many funny stories to me.

In the year of her fifty-fifth birthday, however, several unforeseen circumstances created the stress that was about to change her life. The first was that one of her best friends became ill with a virulent form of pneumonia and died suddenly. Not long thereafter, another one of her cruising pals died as well. These tragic events caused her to look at her own life, and the plans she had made for the future.

The second stressor was when Babs did look at her future, she became aware that although she had a good paying job, much of her compensation was "off the books," and this did not leave her any kind of retirement security. Now she had to consider what she could do to create retirement income.

Babs has three children: two sons and a daughter. Her daughter was married and very established as an attorney in a prestigious Manhattan law firm. Her two sons had followed their father and moved to Southern California to pursue their careers. Every year she would come out to spend time with her boys and, along with her ex-husband, tour the area. For a couple of years, they passed through the same location in which she commented to her ex-husband—who owned an IHOP restaurant—that this would be an excellent location to open another one. He responded to her by saying: "Well if you think it's such a good idea, **why don't you do it**?" She returned to Long Island with that challenge ringing in her ears, but finding every reason why it was not possible for her. His statement, however, created the cognitive dissonance and inner stress to precipitate a major transformation in her life.

Being a very self-motivated person, Babs did not just forget her ex-husband's challenge, or her concern for retirement options, or the pain of losing two of her best girlfriends. With these events being the catalyst, she decided that she could move to California, and create a new life for herself as the owner and manager of a brand new IHOP. All she needed to do was sell her home, move across country and find another home, get the loan for the franchise, have her restaurant built while she did the necessary training, and she'd be good to go. With the courage and determination that make her the kind of woman I described, she accomplished all of these tasks in one year.

Today, she is one of the most successful franchise owners within the IHOP family. Her restaurant is a model for how the company wants their franchises to be run, and she is firmly established and loved as a pillar of the community in Menifee, California. This year she was given an award for going over two million dollars in sales, and she has more plans to expand the restaurant so that customers can sit outside.

Babs is a wonderful example of a person who did not just transplant herself from the east to the west coast, but transformed her entire life by taking the kind of risks that many of us shy away from. She bet on herself and it paid off. She is a model for the possibilities that exist for all of us in later maturity if we believe in ourselves and are capable of making such changes. She did not wait for life and time to turn her dreams into long forgotten memories of something that could have been, but took the risk of personal transformation that is available, to some degree, for all of us.

The fear response in the human brain can also immobilize us from taking these kinds of risks. Many seniors would like to take the chance of creating a better life for themselves, but instead decide to give into their fears and wait for the right time or the right person to help them make a decision. This choice is poignantly characterized by a local writer in her poem titled, *The Particulars of Waiting*:

I am waiting, have been waiting
a long time. Waiting out my childhood,
sitting in my room, an island surrounded
by books, the door closed.
Waiting out winters in my brownstone
when it snowed and you did not come,
never appeared beneath my lighted tree
nor left your footprints
in the new snow on my front steps.
Never came to watch me while I slept
and, therefore, could not wonder
whether it was of you I dreamed.

Waiting out long summers, lazy and laughing
plaiting my hair with tanned hands.
Not knowing when, but still quite sure.
I waited at carnivals and at the ends of piers
and in the last row of pews. Waited, standing
at shop windows, looking past my reflection.
Waited, walking alone through pines.
I was waiting the morning the bathroom light

caught silver at my temple,
the night the lamp cast faint shadows
at the corners of my mouth.

I am waiting now, looking down at my hands,
their patterns of spots and veins.
I have waited, am waiting, will wait.
But will you hurry now, as time
is growing thin and I can hardly make out
the face of the clock in this dim light.
Ricki Mandeville, Silver Birch Press, 2014

I hope that all of us will take the chance to create the lives we want to live rather than waiting and hoping that they will happen on their own.

EXERCISE #3

Transforming the way we see ourselves and creating goals for transformative life change can be a scary process. Even if you like the way your life is now and do not want to initiate any changes, I would like you to work through this exercise as a way of examining all your options. If you do wish to make changes in your life, I hope this gives some clarity to your thoughts and direction for creative action. Remember, you cannot progress toward your goals without stating them clearly and then taking action.

You may want to keep a note pad handy as you go through the visualization in order to write down significant insights.

I would like you to find a quiet place and sit comfortably. . . . Close your eyes and relax. . . . On the screen of your mind project an image of how you would like to be in five years. . . . Where do you live? . . . What do you look like physically? . . . With whom are your most important relationships? . . . How do you feel about yourself? . . . Take some time and allow the image you create to be anything you want. . . . Better health. . . . Improved relationships or a new relationship . . . Weight loss. . . A different living situation.

When you are finished with this visualization, I would like you to get out some notebook paper and answer the following questions:

1. If I were doing what I really wanted to do, what would that look like?

2. What things about myself or my life would I need to change in order to fulfill my goal?

3. What are the objectives I need to create to meet my goal? If you are not sure, try to break it down into baby steps. If you're still not sure, consider who you might consult or what resources you could draw upon to answer the question. Write down three objectives that you can meet in the next 6 months.

4. What are the beliefs and/or judgements that keep me from going after my goals?

5. What do I fear would happen if I made this kind of transformation?

6. What would it take to overcome my fears?

If you are serious about making personal, relationship, or professional changes, it might be helpful to find a good therapist or look for a coach who assists people with making these kinds of life changes.

COMFORT OR CHALLENGE

*They both listened silently to the water, which to them was
not just water, but the
Voice of Life, the voice of Being, of perpetual Becoming.*
                              --Herman Hesse, *Siddhartha*

The years teach much which the days never know.
                              --Ralph Waldo Emerson

One of the secrets of life that emerges from the traditions of the East is that life is a process not unlike the flow of water, and that successful living and aging necessitates moving with the flow (the Tao, the first cause and underlying essence of all), letting it work through and guide one's life. Wholeness is found in taking, like water, the course of least resistance, in relaxing and drifting like a leaf caught in the wind. Aging is most enjoyable when it is graceful rather than abrupt, flowing rather than hesitant. To get our water wings and get into the flow of life requires that we let go of our attachment to the security of the shoreline, which has held the story of our life, and learn to live and move in the present moment. Flowing with life is much like "tubing," that joyful experience of getting an inner tube and just letting a stream or a river carry you along with the current. You don't really have to do anything but enjoy the experience.

To be able to go with the flow requires that we find a harmonious balance between comfort and challenge. Enjoying too much comfort leads to boredom and laziness. On the other hand, too much challenge puts us right back in the same fast lane from which we have just moved. Later maturity gives us the opportunity to enjoy the comfort that comes from not having to compete as much, not having to work as long or hard as we used to, and taking time to enjoy our friends and bask in our new-found freedom from the pressures of parenting. Now we can ask, "What would I like to do with this day?" rather than "What do I have to do today?" This is the comfort of being able to choose how we spend our time, rather than facing the demands that have been so stressful in the past. We can choose to relax and read a book or watch a movie. We can get up and watch the sunrise with a cup of coffee, and later watch the sunset with our favorite herbal tea. Hopefully, we have taken care of our money so that we can live in the comfort that all our hard work now affords us. We can travel to places we only dreamed of before, and spend much more time there, because we don't have a schedule to keep. In more personal terms, we can just be ourselves, without the worry and burden of previous roles and facades. The comfort of later maturity can be analogous to putting on an old pair of slippers that have been worn until they fit just right and feel so good.

What then are the challenges of later maturity? Aren't we just supposed to ease into the sunset of our golden years? Boring! What I would like to suggest is that these years can be the most creative and rewarding years of our lives if we accept the opportunities that are available to us. Learning new skills, meeting new people, enriching our current relationships, expressing our creativity in novel ways and being open to the infinite possibilities of the universe are just some of those challenges. We can never know what direction life will take despite all our goals and plans. The key to creativity is in surrendering to the basic uncertainty of everything, allowing ourselves to appreciate and participate in its beauty. This is the challenge of living in the present, surrendering to what is, and flowing with life through the passage of time. These are the actions that reward us with an active and inquiring mind, a vivacious spirit and a wise and kindly soul. And these actions set our feet firmly on the path that takes us through the landscapes of aging with novelty and wonder.

Perhaps the most daunting challenge of this journey is responding to and connecting with the infinite. "The universal, nonlocal part of the soul is not touched by our actions," writes Deepak Chopra, "but is connected to a spirit that is pure and unchanging. . . Whatever else we are, no matter how much of a mess we may have made of our lives, it is always possible to tap into the part of the soul that is universal, the infinite field of pure potential, and change the course of our destiny."[1] Later maturity is the time to bring about these changes, and, in fact, to embrace change as a way of being. We can all take comfort in the knowledge that relaxing and being open to novelty and change can be one and the same.

Many boomers, however, are faced with physical and emotional challenges that aren't a matter of choice. Some are not able to enjoy the potential comfort or the novel possibilities of later maturity due to a debilitating illness. They are in pain most of the time and have difficulty sleeping or just doing the tasks of everyday living. In fact, chronic conditions and degenerative illnesses have replaced infectious diseases and acute illnesses as the leading cause of death. For those who are sick or in constant pain it is not uncommon to fall victim to depression, or to experience the anxiety that this is all you have to look forward to, or that you don't have much longer to live. For those living alone, as many boomers are, the fear of future setbacks and the advancing of their illness can be as overwhelming as the disease itself. Retreating from friends and loved ones is a real possibility under these circumstances. These factors contribute to what is being reported as a health care crisis in the coming years.

Because Americans are living longer and baby boomers are aging, it is being predicted that the population aged 65 years and older will double in the next 25 years. In 2030, when the last of the baby boomers turn 65, approximately 20% of Americans will be older adults. The Center for Disease Control and Prevention (CDC) reports that two out of every three older Americans have multiple chronic conditions and their treatment will account for 66% of the country's health care budget. Chronic conditions include Alzheimer's disease, diabetes, various forms of heart disease, COPD, and a host of other illnesses.

While the country prepares for the "silver tsunami" of physical problems, mental problems are also on the rise. The CDC also reports that one in four seniors has some type of mental health problem, such as a mood disorder not associated with normal aging. Although social contact and support is a strong predictor of well-being, a substantial number of seniors report that they do not get the social and emotional support they need. Further, we know that mental health problems can exacerbate physical conditions, as those with mental health issues tend to smoke and use alcohol more, do not eat properly, exercise less, and in general show significant deficits in self-care.[2]

If you are not sick or depressed by now, I'd like to present some images of challenges—through interviews and current movie reviews—that many boomers may face along the journey of aging. The significance of these examples is not in the challenges themselves, but in how they were met and the subsequent outcome.

At 52 years of age, Bob is a younger boomer who has already faced many challenges. Eleven years after the marriage to his first wife, her repeated affairs caused him to ask her to leave, even though they had four children at home aged 3, 5, 8 and 12. So at 37, Bob was a single parent to four young children, an ex-wife who moved away and refused to help with parenting, and no family member to turn to for support and help. He was forced to sell his home and find something with a more affordable mortgage. Uprooted, he faced the prospect of raising four young children on his own, as he looked to change careers to make more money and give him more time to be with his kids.

Bob had worked in sales and owned a small business with a partner who cheated him out of much of the revenue. Now he decided to embark on a new career as a financial planner. His timing wasn't ideal: following the famous Y2K panic, the stock market went down for the following three years, his manager quit, and the office where he was employed fell into total disarray. Despite being named "rookie of the year," Bob felt like a "pinball," as he constantly bounced from one school to another to pick up his children. Through all of this, he stuck with his initial plan, and got his Series 7 license. He passed the test, which has an 80% fail rate, on his first attempt.

Despite how well he seemed to be doing, things in his field were unstable and Bob found himself jobless. That went on for a year. While he looked for a new position, Bob did some day trading with mixed results. In 2008, he decided to work as a sales representative, earning 48k, which wasn't enough to support his family. He figured it would at least help to pay the mounting bills while he looked for something better.

Finally, through his long association with a Christian Businessman's Association, most of the time as their president, another member referred him to a local credit union with a religious affiliation. He negotiated a deal with the credit union president to start his own financial planning company with an office in their building, and settled into the career in which he now thrives.

Having worked through the turmoil of his 30s and 40s, Bob is on the verge of buying a much larger wealth management firm, with several offices and numerous employees under his supervision. His three older children are all in college and living independently, while his youngest son is still at home. But he is up for these challenges, having learned much from his former successes and failures, and never giving up his belief in himself.

The boomer generation has faced more challenges and enjoyed less stability than the generations that came before them. Members of prior generations tended to stay in the same job for a lifetime and retire at 65. People also tended to remain in marriages and were not as often traumatized by bitter divorces. When I said that boomers need to embrace change as a continuous way of life, I was thinking of many of my clients who have been down-sized, outsized, riffed, and otherwise treated unfairly in the business world. Some of these same people have suffered through adulterous relationships or have had one or more painful divorces. The question that we must ask ourselves is never why me? It is always what can I do now?

Bob is an example of a person who has faced some severe challenges and has not given into self-pity or regret. He has chosen to seize the moment and create a new life for himself and his children. I am honored to call him my friend.

Many movies over the past few years have targeted a boomer audience. In 2015, *Learning to Drive* and *The Intern*, focused on the lives of boomers as they reach their 60s and 70s.

Learning to Drive, opens with protagonist Wendy (Patricia Clarkson), a middle-aged boomer, jumping into a New York City cab in which her husband has tried to make a getaway after letting her know over dinner that he is planning on leaving her. While she cries and rants and flails at Ted (Jake Weber), the cabdriver Darwan, played by Ben Kingsley, quietly listens and watches in the rear-view mirror. Ted, unpersuaded, exits the cab and Darwan must drive Wendy home alone.

Thus begins a little slice of life movie featuring two of America's better actors. Their different cultural backgrounds add up to different kinds of challenges. Darwan is a Sikh who has secured political asylum, and now lives in a cramped basement flat in Queens with several other Indian men. He teaches driving by day and drives a cab at night. Wendy is a literary critic and lifelong New Yorker who has never learned to drive.

While Wendy faces the crisis of divorce and struggles to regain her independence, Darwan is being asked to accept an arranged marriage with a woman from India. His new bride, Jasleen, has just arrived in America and is completely overwhelmed with her new life. Wendy needs to learn how to live life on her own and acquire the skills that she had previously relied on her husband for. Darwan is filled with anxiety about making a new relationship work.

Together they form a team of teacher and student, the lesson of learning to drive filled with metaphors about life: be aware of your surroundings, start moving ahead, learn to control your anger, and always know where you are going. Although there are hints of romance in their relationship, what develops is a platonic bond that gives strength and courage to both.

Learning to Drive is a heartfelt movie about starting over and starting anew—tasks with which we boomers can all relate.

The Intern also features two outstanding actors, Robert De Niro and Anne Hathaway, in a comedy about what happens when different generations must interact in a rapidly changing business environment. Ben (De Niro) is a retired widower who applies for and is accepted for a senior internship program at an online women's fashion shopping network. Jules (Hathaway) is its CEO. At first, Jules doesn't perceive any need for an intern and is certainly in no mood for an elder's advice. But once Ben is assigned to her exclusively, his calm and patient demeanor provides a valuable balance to her stressed-out impatience.

There are plenty of humorous generational issues: Ben's trouble setting up a Facebook account, the dating problems and sloppy dress of the office millennials, the shock when these same millennials see Ben with a briefcase and treat it like an antique, while they take for granted Jules riding her bike through the office. But in the end their humanity comes through.

Ben is lonely and needs to fill the hole in his life since the death of his wife. Jules has great conflict about how to balance her time and attention to work, with time to be at home with her househusband Matt and their precocious daughter Paige. As in *The Driving Lesson*, the relationship between the two main characters turns into a friendship that benefits both. Jules is able to learn from Ben's years of management and life experience, and Ben is able to recognize the brilliance of Jules' leadership and support her decision making. In an ideal world, this would be the way boomers and millennials would interact in the workplace.

However, evidence does not show this to be true. The research shows, as I have stated before, that interactions between these generations are often marked with conflict. If boomers could only show the patience and good will that Ben shows in this movie, then perhaps after a time, younger workers might be ready to listen to their advice and welcome their years of experience.

I enjoyed these movies and would recommend that you stream them through whatever service you use. There were no explosions, car chases, or bullets fired. They are just movies about human beings facing challenges that are both thought provoking and endearing.

A final interview illustrates how even a severe physical challenge can be met and overcome with the right attitude.

I sat in Tom's living room on a comfortable couch, while he sat in his wheelchair, leaning forward and twisting from time to time to try to reduce the pain in his back and buttocks. Tom is a leading-edge boomer who contracted poliomyelitis (also called Infantile Paralysis, because it affected so many young children) at age four, during one of the summer epidemics that struck the United States prior to the vaccine developed in the mid-fifties.

The result was post-polio paralysis, and now, later in life, a second blow with the post-polio syndrome that can affect polio survivors later in life and cause new and significant symptoms.

Tom told me how at age four he suffered from a two-week illness with fevers of 104 and 105 degrees. Once admitted to Los Angeles General Hospital and given the diagnosis of polio, Tom kept walking in his crib hoping that would stave off the paralysis that he knew, even at age four, often happens following the virus. His nurses kept telling him to lie still, and he only did so once he had become too ill to do anything else. When he finally awakened after days of sleeping with little or no awareness of what was going on around him, he found himself paralyzed from the neck down. He could barely move his fingers across his chest. He later wrote in his poem, *July 1948*, "He can only move his fingers./ Only a little./ Only to crawl his hands across his chest/ to scratch his nose." Breathing was so labored and impaired that he came within several hours of being put in an iron lung. After surviving the acute phase of his illness, he was moved to Orthopedic Hospital, a rehab facility that cared for many post-polio children. There he fought his paralysis, working to regain strength, while being distressed with his hospitalized and separation from his mother. As this was the late 1940s, the treatment he received was rudimentary, and, in his words, "well-intentioned but relatively inhumane."

Because of the neuroplasticity of motor neurons in the central peripheral nervous system, surviving motor neurons sent out connections that bypassed and took over for those that had been destroyed. Consequently, Tom regained strength, especially in his upper body, and was eventually able to walk again with the help of orthopedic leg braces and cuffed arm crutches (in those days called Kinney Sticks after Sister Kinney who designed them and was a pioneer in the treatment of post-polio). After years of walking on those crutches, he suffered considerable muscle damage and pain in his shoulders and elbows, and was forced to use a wheelchair like the one that he is sitting in as he faces me now. He is a brilliant man, with large hands and an intense gaze that takes in everything as I listen to the story of his illness with few questions needed. His upper body is well developed, but due to paralysis, the growth of his legs was stunted. We both agree that he might have been 6'4" had it not been for that illness.

After attending elementary and secondary schools for the disabled, Tom graduated from a mainstream high school of mostly able-bodied students and then went to a small, very selective liberal arts college. Some years later, he returned to academia and received a Master's Degree in Social Psychology at Cal State University, Los Angeles, and eventually was awarded a PhD in Clinical Psychology from the University of Houston, specializing in somatopsychology (also known as rehab psychology). Not wanting to take the comfortable path, he accomplished all these milestones without using any of the help offered those with disabilities, such as handicapped parking, or assistance with notes and test taking. With this educational background, he went on to treat disabled veterans, supervise disabled students at two universities and became a professor at University of La Verne.

Tom states boldly that his biggest challenge was in accepting and "making friends" with his emotions, spending some years in therapy with a local clinician. Because he suffers from the late-onset effects of post-polio syndrome, including chronic fatigue type symptoms, increased muscle weakness, and pain derived both from overuse of upper body muscles and from sitting in a wheelchair for so many years, he realizes that "aging with polio is my form of aging."

To say that Tom has a strong and determined personality and has overcome many challenges is certainly an understatement. He is a man who has accepted himself in ways that many of us never do, and has not allowed his disability to keep him from a full and satisfying life. He is a boomer who has made the second half of life a time for creative endeavors—teaching and supervising students, writing essays and some very powerful poetry, and pursuing his goal of authoring a book on coping with disability. Most of all, he is an example of how to handle challenges in a courageous and creative way, and an inspiration to any boomer whose challenges may be different but equally daunting.

Whether we choose to enjoy a more comfortable second half of life, seek new challenges, or continue to face our own specific challenges in a positive way, the important thing to realize is that the choice is ours to make. Finding the right balance of comfort and challenge is one of the keys to making later maturity a rewarding time of life.

EXERCISE #4

One thing that keeps us from finding a harmonious balance between comfort and challenge is that we are stuck in the past because of regrets—regrets about squandered opportunities, impulsive acts, about not being the best parent, about a painful divorce and its results on family and children, or maybe an affair. Many boomers with whom I had the pleasure of working with, felt that they let their lives slip away without really living, while others remained stuck in past negativity.

How can we move on with our lives? I think that awareness of the problem and then adopting a different point of view regarding the outcome can be very helpful. I am going to include resentments, for they also trap you in the past and keep you from living in the present moment.

I would like you to take out a piece of white paper and divide it into four equal parts. In the upper left part of the paper write the word "regrets." Now go to the upper right side and write the word "resentments." Continue to the bottom left and write "appreciation," and in the bottom right corner write "gratitude."

Remember that in this exercise we are working with corresponding words from the diagonal corners. Start in the upper left quadrant and write out all the decisions you made, actions you took or wish you had taken, everything about your life you regret. Start each sentence with "I regret" and add some detail about why this has caused you to feel that way. When you are finished, go to the lower right quadrant and rewrite each sentence, substituting "I am grateful" where I regret was. Explain how you can be grateful for something for which you only felt regret before. You might say something like, "I am grateful for my divorce because I found someone I really love, and the kids love him/her as well." Or perhaps where there still is a lot of pain, "I am grateful for the time we had together despite the pain of our divorce." In the case of a bad decision it might be something like, "I am grateful for the decision I made, because it brought about a valuable life lesson." Letting go of regrets and resentments can be very difficult, because each time we think about them, we reinforce the brain's habitual patterns. We need, therefore, to change the way our brain processes this old information by presenting new insight and then repeating it over and over. Repetition is the key to changing the way you think. Let your inner wisdom guide you in seeing your regrets and resentments in a new light.

Now repeat this process with the quadrants that have the words "resent" and "appreciate" in the respective corners. You might have written, "I resent your nagging," and you can change it to something like, "I appreciate your reminders, for they help me get things done." Or it may be "I resent my boss," and this can change to "I appreciate that you were tough on me, for it helped me to be a better employee."

Your page should look something like this:

Regrets   Resentments

Appreciation   Gratitude

When you are finished with your sentences, notice how the diagonal sides present two different perspectives on the same issue. A positive side can be found for most of the negative experiences and negative relationships in our lives if we look for it.

If you are inspired to let go of some regrets or resentments, I suggest you write a good-bye letter to each one stating why you have held onto it for so long, how it has benefited you, and that you are finally ready to let it go. Because this is a letter, finish it with the declaration "good bye" and sign your name. You may want to keep this letter or take it to your shredder. It is your letter, so do whatever you feel is right.

P.S. This is another good use of your journal.

THEY'RE ONLY MEMORIES

To be alive is to have a past. Our only choice is whether we will repress or re-create the past. Childhood may be distant, but it is never quite lost; as full grown men and women we carry tiny laughing and whimpering children around inside us. We either repress the past and continue to fight its wars with new personnel or we invite it into awareness so that we may see how it has shaped the present.

--Sam Keen, *Your Mythic Journey*

This is my thirty-seventh year as a psychotherapist, and I have treated thousands of people, many of those in the stage of life I am now calling later maturity. One experience my clients all have in common is that they are feeling a great deal of emotional pain. I usually start by asking what brings them to my office and they begin to tell the story that is their life or some significant part of it. As they tell me of the recent events that have brought them to this specific moment, I inquire about earlier experiences, and we go further back into their pasts. To fully understand the problems they face, I must get an understanding of where they have been, their life experience, the traumas and triumphs that constitute their story.

What I most often find is that, though my clients may track the beginning of their problems to more recent challenges, the roots of their suffering are in events that happened many years before. More than that, they are suffering from the negative beliefs these events engendered, often without awareness of their cause. As we move into the second half of life, I think we are more determined than ever not to keep living exactly as we have lived, under the influence of the same fears and hindrances that have kept us from fulfillment in the past. It may be harder than ever to accept that even 50, or 60, or 70 years into this life, we continue to repeat the past, or live out patterns of behavior established in our earlier years. Once we recognize it, we may face the sinking feeling that no matter what we do, we can never be free of the past's powerful grip.

Unless we've done a fair amount of introspection, either in therapy or on our own, we may not be consciously aware that the way we react to others now is the result of conditioning in childhood. Even when we understand this in an objective way, it's very hard to look at the ways our core beliefs about ourselves, the world, relationships, success and failure have also been conditioned in childhood. To fully recognize that you are reacting to your wife or husband with the beliefs and responses of an eight-year-old is difficult to accept. But that is often the case. Are we doomed or is Keen right that we still are able to "re-create the past" in the way we currently live our lives? When the past is repressed, it comes out in the present in the form of transference. This happens when we unconsciously see our parent's face, or the face of another significant adult, in the face of someone in the present, when we hear our parent's words rather than the words currently being spoken. And because our brains interpret the information our senses pick up, it is possible to re-live our past in the present, never knowing that we are completely out of sequence in terms of person, place or time. We see and hear with our senses but we interpret what we see and what we hear instantaneously through the filters of our past. We are never completely free from transference, but we can become more aware of it. A friend of mine tells me that she sometimes says to her husband in the heat of an argument, "How old are you right now, because I feel about four years old." He'll respond, "Twelve, I guess I'm about twelve." Then they both laugh and consider their current situation from a cleaner, more present day perspective.

David Richo writes in *When the Past is Present*, "Transference is an unconscious displacement of feelings, attitudes, expectations, perceptions, reactions, beliefs, and judgments that were appropriate to former figures in our lives, mostly parents, onto people in the present."[1] So then, if transference is such a powerful force, why have I titled this chapter "They're Only Memories"? Because, it is important to recognize that the hurts and wounds of childhood, just like the hurts and wounds of former relationships, ultimately only exist in the form of memories, which we can acknowledge as belonging to the past. Only by consciously separating past from present can we free ourselves from ingrained and repetitive behaviors and reactions.

This kind of conscious change can be a daunting task. The problem is threefold. One, these bits of information lie in the subconscious, and out of our immediate awareness. In terms of neurological processing abilities, the subconscious mind is millions of times more powerful than the conscious mind. Cellular biologist Bruce Lipton, in *The Biology of Belief,* reports that the subconscious mind can process 20,000,000 environmental stimuli per second in contrast to the 40 environmental stimuli the conscious mind can process in the same second. Two, when activated by a perceived "threat," the subconscious mind reacts before we can think it through consciously. The brain's reaction to this threat, whether perceived or real, is to activate the stress response, or what we commonly call the flight-or-fight response. This automatic response can take the form of physical action or behavioral reactions, which have been conditioned in childhood. "The fundamental behaviors, beliefs and attitudes we observe in our parents," writes Lipton, "become 'hard-wired' as synaptic pathways in our subconscious minds. Once programed into the subconscious mind, they control our biology for the rest of our lives . . . unless we can figure out a way to reprogram them." He goes on to speak to the verbal abuses of parents and other authority figures in stating, "These verbal abuses become defined as 'truths' that unconsciously shape the behavior and potential of the child throughout life."[2] Unfortunately then, the stress response can be turned on by anything that triggers a memory of an unhappy or traumatic past event, and the repetitive turning on and off this response, eventually leads to both physical and emotional problems. And finally, even though they are seriously outdated and flawed, we hold onto these previously conditioned attitudes and beliefs because they *seem* to comprise our identity; we think that our *story* is who we truly *are*.

The truth is that even when the negative and limiting beliefs about the world and other people, and the way we automatically react when "our buttons are pushed," no longer serve us well, it can be more comfortable to hold onto a distorted belief than to experience the anxiety created by the possibility of change. Even if those distorted beliefs and behavior patterns have damaged our relationships, led to failure in our professional lives, and seem inextricably intertwined with our anxiety or depression, changing them can feel scarier than living with the familiar.

Regardless of the inherent difficulties, I am issuing a challenge to all of us in this stage of life to activate the courage needed to face those left-over heartaches from the past, to create a method to work through the feelings and beliefs still attached to them, and to learn to let go of them so that we can get on with our lives. When this is done, it is possible to re-experience these memories as just that: only memories that need not have power over us anymore. We can learn to reflect upon our history as just events, events that no longer carry the hurt and anger they once did. Dr. Dan Siegel, Executive Director of the Mindsight Institute, states, "When unresolved issues are writing our life story, we are not our own autobiographers; we are merely recorders of how the past continues, often without our awareness, to intrude upon our present experience and shape our future directions."[3]

To give you an idea of how the past can continue to intrude upon a person's present experience, let me recount to you my own story. I was a ten- year-old boy, about to experience the major trauma of my childhood.

I grew up with an angry father, who might now be regarded as abusive. He used switches and his belt to keep me terrified of him and willing to do whatever he said. My mother, much younger than he, forged her own form of escape through prescription drugs which she surreptitiously parceled out from her own mother-in-law's supply. My grandmother was registered as addicted to codeine for migraine headaches, and my mother regularly pilfered part of these drugs to cope with her own emotional pain. It was only much later I learned that when my sister and I were dropped off at the local five and dime it was to give my mother the time she needed to take part of the codeine, which came in small packets of powder, for herself. When the drugs weren't enough, our mom attempted suicide by pulling an electric radio into her bath.

The details remain vivid. It was the summer of my tenth year. Things weren't going well for my family, but that wasn't unusual. We were struggling to survive financially. My dad, who worked as an airplane mechanic for Lockheed, had just recently found out that my mother had spent most of the money in the bank to pay for the extra prescriptions now needed to make up for what she had taken. Violent arguments and incriminations followed his discovery, as well as a litter of torn check stubs that I can still see strewn across the floor. I didn't exactly know what all of this meant, but I knew it was bad, and I was scared to death of what might come. Then, on a Friday afternoon, at about 4:30 or so, my mother went in to take a bath. This, in itself, was unusual for her because my father would return from work at about 5:00, and normally she would have been preparing dinner. That time of day was already electric with tension and laden with anxiety for me, because my dad's arrival often meant sudden and unpredictable fury if I hadn't done just what he had ordered before leaving that morning. But that day's electricity was destined for a different purpose, for out of desperation, anger, and vindictiveness, my mother was preparing to pull our little Zenith table radio into the tub to electrocute herself. I guess she intended the message for my father as a way of punishing him, to make him blame himself and feel responsible for her death, but I got a host of mordant messages that day, that have haunted me ever since: messages about love and relationships, about money, and about my worthiness as a person. I could go on at length about the negative beliefs that were formed that day, but I've gotten ahead of myself.

An ominous sense of apprehension began to fill me as my dad came into the house and asked about my mother's whereabouts. I don't remember whether my sister or I told him, but I do remember him calling for her at the bathroom door. When she did not respond, fear gripped me. As fate would have it, the knob on the outside of that door, like many things in that awful house where I grew up, was broken. As he pounded and yelled, I ran from the house into the yard. In utter terror, I waited, just as I was to wait many other times when life and death hung in the balance for my mother, trying not to think about what was happening behind that bathroom door. Whatever force pulled me back inside my house remains a mystery, but I knew I had to go back in.

When I got into the house again, I saw my mother stretched out in the living room and my father desperately trying to revive her. My father looked up at me with that same fire I had seen so many times in his eyes, and spat out, "Where the hell have you been?" My mind raced, my heart thundered. I had no answer. I snapped out of it instantly as my dad yelled at me to go to the neighbors' house and phone for an ambulance, something I had never done before. In fact, I'd only used a phone on one other occasion. Remember, those were not the days when most ten-year-old's carried their own cell phones. Those were the days when having a phone in your house was a luxury, not the necessity it is today, and we were too poor to have one. Now I had to run down the street to make that horrible call. And run I did, frantically, the half block to the only friendly neighbors we had, where I asked politely to use their phone and attempted to get somebody to send an ambulance to our house. Because my voice was obviously that of a young boy, the operator refused to believe me and asked for an adult. I put the phone down wondering if my mother would die because of my delay. Knowing that I had failed, I had to run back and face my father for a second time.

I ran back to the same terrifying scene of my father attempting CPR and my sister kneeling silently alongside, and tried to explain what had happened. "You get back there," my dad screamed, "and get that ambulance here." I flew back to the neighbor's house, my heart pounding in my ears. I didn't know if I was more afraid of my mother dying on the living room floor or my father waiting to kill me if I failed again. When I arrived, breathless and dripping sweat, my neighbors caught me in flight, telling me that they had vouched for me with the operator and an ambulance was on its way. I still remember my sweet neighbor, in her southern drawl saying, "If that boy says it happened, **then** it happened!"

After a flurry of questions about what had happened, how it happened, and whether she was alive or not, none of which I could answer, I again turned and ran home. My mind raced with these new questions, giving shape to vague impressions I already had, and my ears rang with the whine of sirens as an ambulance mercifully pulled in front of the chain link fence that separated our house from the rest of the neighborhood, and in fact, the rest of the world.

Where were our Dobermans and why weren't they barking? The dogs that made our yard feel so dangerous to the rest of the neighborhood had been put in the garage, I guess by my sister. I waited at the gate while the paramedics went in, followed them and hovered over and around my mother while they tended to her, asking my father questions, the answers to which I don't remember hearing. I was either too stunned to hear his answers or have blocked those memories out. Finally, I saw them wrap her in a blanket, strap her to a stretcher, and put her into the ambulance. Not one tear had come from my eyes. I didn't really know what had happened or what would happen, but I knew my mother was miraculously alive. I couldn't speak. I was afraid to look at anybody, lest they see my weakness, my fear, and the emerging feelings that if my mother could abandon me in this way, did she really love me after all? Once in the back yard again, my sister covered her face and cried out, "she tried to kill herself," and the answers to all my questions crystallized around that shocking declaration. I stood alone in the shadows of the house and felt an intense pain that I could not fully understand.

My mother lived that day, but this event changed the lives of a then ten- year-old boy and his thirteen-year-old sister in ways that are still being made evident as they live on into their seventies. Through the rest of my childhood and adolescence, I lived in constant fear that my mother would try it again. That night, when my father and sister and I went to see her in the hospital, my mother called me to her bedside and whispered in my ear, "What floor are we on?" I thought that she was going to reassure me that things were ok and that she would not try to kill herself again. Instead she said something which only intensified the fears that had been building for many years. The message I got was, "I'm not sorry and I'm not sure I won't try it again." Luckily, the tiny hospital in Northridge had only one floor, but I knew what she meant. I never told my sister or my father of my mother's request that evening, but it is another trauma that scarred me deeply. When she came home I would check the number of razor blades in the drawer after every time she used the bathroom. As I grew older and would go out at night, I always came home early so that I could be there if there was another suicide attempt. Though the failure of this first attempt seemed to take all the steam out of her desperation, at least for a while, it in no way reduced the anxiety that I had experienced through most of my childhood and adolescence, and experience at lesser levels to this day. Long before this trauma, I was frightened by the constant arguments between my mother and father, the violent fist fights my father had with his brother, Ralph, and the rage that filled my father's eyes when he was angry with me or when he would whip me. I grew up in a home addicted to violence and I was always afraid that someone, maybe even I, would be killed. My fears—and consequent feelings of responsibility for my mother—continued until the day, when out of a different kind of desperation, that of pain and illness, she successfully completed that which she had begun nineteen years earlier.

My sister met me at the door of our old home and told me that our mother, now 52 years old, had indeed, committed suicide. This time she had made sure she wouldn't fail; she had used a razor blade, taken pills and turned on the gas. As she was still living with my father, she scribbled a final note for him: "Can you ever forgive me?" was all it said. She left no note for my sister and me. My mother's suicide, like most suicides, laid waste to the family she left behind.

Despite my mother's first suicide attempt, my father's rage and violence, and other associated traumas that came later in our childhoods, my sister and I, bearing the wounds of our dysfunctional family, grew into adulthood. I married at 23—far too young for me—hoping to escape some of the demons of anxiety and depression that followed me. My mistrust of women, my fear that any woman I loved would, in some way, leave me, and my belief that I really didn't deserve love played havoc with our relationship, all contributing to the dissolution of our marriage after 15 tumultuous years. However, two very important and life-altering events happened: the birth of my son and many years of serious therapy.

Being in weekly individual and group therapy with an excellent therapist helped me to confront my fears, learn how to manage my depression, and start to understand myself for the first time. I began to integrate all the painful experiences of my childhood, learned to take responsibility for the problems that were mine, and let go of those that belonged to someone else. I never dreamed that a decade later, I would become a therapist myself.

My son's arrival opened a place in my heart that had long been closed, a place of love and vulnerability that is impossible to describe. When my son Wesley came gently into my life, it was never to be the same. Just to hold him in my arms was the best thing that had ever happened to me and I was determined not to be the same kind of father that I had experienced growing up.

When the loving family I thought I had finally created, ended in a bitter divorce after fifteen years, I carried on as a single parent, managing the pressure of a professional practice. When Wesley left home for college, I lost my sense of purpose; I felt overwhelmed by what's commonly referred to as the *empty nest syndrome*, a condition which usually describes the reaction of mothers. At the same time, my professional life was in disarray, as the changes in reimbursement policies for mental health care had led to a devastating loss of income and, with it, a decline in self-esteem. Despite all my years of therapy, all the years of feeling that I had overcome or at least understood the impact of my childhood, I fell into a deep depression. A year after I'd recovered and returned to work, I was diagnosed with cancer. These are the kinds of events that hit us all as we age; few of us are immune to loss and change. Through these life events I was aware of the presence of the negative beliefs and self-limiting patterns that had begun in my childhood. I saw clearly the belief that I didn't deserve good things and would avoid or just give up in the face of a strong challenge. I was aware of a deep fear that something would happen to my son or that I would lose him in some awful way. I carried with me many other painful memories, as well as fears about the future, but I was also aware of how I could use various therapeutic techniques to continue the process of letting go, and create new patterns and beliefs to bring back the joy and fulfillment that I was missing.

For many of us, later maturity can provide the opportunity to become our own autobiographers, to write our life stories in the way we want them to be, not merely allowing them to be written by the conditioning of the past. The writing can be in the form of a life review, personal memoir, or commitment to the desires of our heart for the remaining time we have left on this earth. This is a time for writing and reflection, for "letting go of things" and painful memories that keep us trapped by the energy we give them, and to be receptive to the myriad possibilities of our present.

Years ago, I watched a rescue of two girls from the high tops of trees that were being engulfed by flood waters. The trees' uppermost branches were only about five feet above the water. Men piloting outboard motor boats tried to position themselves to be able to catch the girls if they jumped, but this required that they let go. They were terribly frightened, and all the rescuers' encouragement could not get them to release the branches to which they clung. Eventually, the children's bus driver, who had been trapped in the trees as well, found a way to get to the girls and pry their fingers free. Each one in turn was swept into the waiting arms of the men in the boats. Finally, the bus driver was also rescued in this same way, so that all three were saved in what could have been a real tragedy.

Sometimes finding our true selves requires facing our worst fears and letting go of what we think of as security. Sometimes enjoying our lives requires asking for and accepting rescue from the things that hold us back. Remember: *they're only memories*; they can't hurt you anymore unless you allow them the power to do so.

EXERCISE #5

Letting go of the past can be a painful experience and you may need a professional therapist to help you with this. Try the following exercise to see if you have buried a lot of your past, or if your childhood has more unpleasant than pleasant memories.

Draw a detailed floor plan of the house of your earliest memory. Take your time and draw all the rooms and perhaps even the yard if you can remember.

1. As you enter each room imagine the events you associate with the room. See if you can remember how it felt to be in that room, what was on the walls, and the furniture that was there.

2. Who lived in that house with you? What do you remember most about those people?

3. What is your happiest memory of that house and that time?

4. What is the most painful memory?

5. What was the overall mood in that household?

6. Which rooms are you unable to remember? Why do you think you are having difficulty remembering these rooms?

7. Are there rooms that you are afraid to enter? Why?

8. Did you have a secret hiding place?

If you find yourself feeling overwhelmed, anxious, or depressed as you do this exercise, please turn to a close friend or a professional for their support and guidance.

ACQUIRING OR DOWNSIZING

The best thing about getting old is that all those things you couldn't have when you were young, you no longer want.

--L.S. McCandless

Then youth itself, though in another dress,
Age is opportunity no less,
And as the evening twilight fades away,
The sky is filled with stars, invisible by day.
--Henry Wadsworth Longfellow, *Morituri Salatumus*

Recently, I was driving along the freeway, minding my own business, when a huge recreational vehicle blew by me in the fast lane. You'll remember that I had chosen to move out of the fast lane some time ago, to pull over and let the younger generation move at the faster pace. Well, I saw that the driver was a senior, as was his wife, and that attached to the back of their RV was another vehicle. In addition, there were bikes and other toys piled up in a storage compartment. I didn't know whether to feel jealous or sorry for the occupants of that home on wheels. But it triggered more thinking about the aging process, and wondering whether it was better to acquire things later in life, when perhaps you could more readily afford them, or to start the process of downsizing to correlate with later maturity. I think everybody in this culture knows the details of acquisition, as we Americans do it so well. But downsizing is another matter entirely, for this means letting go of the things we have acquired, and beyond that, letting go of the concept of acquiring altogether.

Anyone familiar with the material of comedian George Carlin, knows that he had a whole routine based on people's "stuff;" how we get it, how we move it, and just what we do with it. It's very clear that he's poking fun at all of us when he implies that the meaning of life is "trying to find a place for your stuff," and that there is a "whole industry based on having to keep an eye on your stuff." But my favorite line concerns the value we put on the stuff that we have collected over the years when he quips, "have you ever noticed that their stuff is shit and your shit is stuff?"

Though not as humorous as the thoughts of George Carlin, my experience with the "stuff" I had accumulated was a traumatic type of downsizing that some of you may be familiar with—forced downsizing. The second half of the 90's played havoc with my career. This was the time in health care reform when managed care was sweeping the country. For those of us in the field of mental health this meant significant changes in the way clients found us, how we delivered our services, and the way we were paid. Most of my colleagues were scrambling to be approved providers for as many HMOs as they could find. Some were thinking of leaving the state of California, retiring early, or considering new careers. Hospitals were finding it hard to compete and many simply closed their doors and sold the property.

It was too early for me to retire, and I had no thoughts of moving out of state, so I was faced with a real dilemma. A large part of my income came from a local psychiatric hospital, for which I did daily group therapy, and held a position which gave me a monthly stipend. I also sat on the Medical Executive Committee, giving me access to all the bad news about the financial situation of the hospital. Every several weeks the hospital administrator called me into his office to inform me that my stipend was reduced by 50% as was the reimbursement for my daily groups. You can only cut things in half for so long, and eventually my income at the hospital was reduced by 85%. I was forced to leave and look for another source of income, in a field decimated by managed care. In desperation, I took a job in a related health care field, grew to hate it in one month, and quickly resigned.

The following several years were no better for me financially or emotionally. I put the house I was living in up for sale and it sat empty for eight months until it finally sold. I had to take money out of my son's college fund just to pay my bills. I thought I might have to file for bankruptcy. My son was attending college in Northern California at that time, and I didn't hear from him all that often, adding to the pain I felt. As was my lifelong pattern, I did not ask anybody for help or advice. I tried to work through this crisis on my own, with unfavorable results. To say I was depressed would be an understatement. I felt devastated and alone. I was overwhelmed with fear and withdrew into a private world of sleep to mask my feelings. One of the saddest parts of this experience was that I felt that I didn't deserve the money I had previously been making, that I had reached for more than I was worth, and now was paying the price. I was reminded at that time of something my mother used to say: "Pride cometh before a fall."

It took me about five years to work through the losses I had suffered and stabilize myself financially and emotionally. I now live in the house that once was my rental, and I'm glad to have it. What I learned during that time was that "things" matter very little in life—what matters is the love and support of friends and family. I was forced to let go of much of the stuff that I accumulated when I was doing well financially, and I am glad for it. Forced to downsize, I have less to worry about, and that was a very important factor in my decision to retire. I no longer feel tied to my possessions, and that brings a sense of relief and a new sense of freedom.

I'm not suggesting that we don't earn as much as we possibly can, just that it's important not to get caught up in the consumerism of our world.

To put my own experience into a theoretical perspective, I'm going to turn to one of my idols in the field of psychology: Swiss psychiatrist and founder of analytical psychology, Carl Gustav Jung. Reprising Jung, life is divided into two halves. The first half is characterized by expansion and adaptation to outer realities, learning how to take hold of life and get along in the world. The tasks for this half are establishing personal identity and independence from our family of origin, establishing adult relationships which may include marriage and starting a family, and utilizing one's abilities in work and society. Eventually, we all cross over into the second half of life, tackling new developmental tasks as previously undeveloped life qualities take on new importance. During the second half of life a person begins to move away from his or her preoccupation with acquisition and external realities and experience an "initiation into the inner reality" as Jung states. There is a gradual shift in attention from things outside oneself to the inner world, a need for deeper self-knowledge and awareness of where each one of us fits in the scheme of creation. Home, then, becomes more than just a place to store our stuff while we go out and look for more stuff, it is the starting place for letting go of the things we have accumulated during the first half of life, to be able to expand our consciousness and look for the deeper meanings.

In both a practical and psychological sense, I'm in agreement with Jung. Later maturity, as I see it, is a time for getting our house in order; for getting rid of things we no longer need, simplifying our lives and focusing on what's most important. When I was in college, my anthropology professor, Dr. Carpenter, told us many stories of the indigenous people of the Artic regions of Canada and Alaska, those whom he studied and worked with in his time away from the classroom. The story that stuck with me over the years concerned their carvings in ivory. He reported that with each new carving, the artist called out to the ivory, asking what shape or animal needed to come out of it. In their carvings, every artist worked to free their subject from the ivory itself. When an igloo, or a whale, or sea lion finally emerged, their work was finished and, since it was the work that was most significant, rather than the object they had created, they just threw away the finished product. Only when outside sources began to influence the Inuit (formerly called Eskimos), did they realize that their carvings could be sold as scrimshaw, that the finished products had value. Eventually, the artists' joy in freeing the spirit of a walrus or a polar bear from the ivory lost its meaning. What replaced it was a new industry based on making money through the sale of scrimshaw. I know that many of you will think that it was a good thing for the Inuit to participate in a free economy system, but for Dr. Carpenter it was very sad. He saw that in learning our ways, they lost their innocence and *joie de vivre*.

What this says to me is that later maturity is our time to let go of the need for stuff, to stop acquiring more and more things, and to start learning to travel light. If the things that we acquire no longer bring us, or our family joy, then it is time to get rid of them. It is time to overcome the hoarding compulsion that so many of us experience, time to give things away or sell them at yard sales, time to feel the lightness that comes from being less encumbered with possessions. Try it; you just might like it.

EXERCISE #6

Find a comfortable chair to sit in or get comfortable in the chair in which you are currently sitting. Take a few minutes to get in touch with your breathing. Focus on the intake and exhalation of your breath. When you are feeling relaxed, create on the screen of your mind a giant yard sale at which you can sell personal items, personal characteristics and habits, and even personal acquaintances.

1. How much of your "stuff" would you put out for sale?

2. Are there things you have been holding onto for too long?

3. Are there personal habits, like smoking or drinking, that you would like to get rid of?

4. What characteristics could go on sale for better upgrades?

5. What fears keep you from letting go of that which does not serve you well anymore?

6. Are there friends or acquaintances who take more than they give?

7. Can you see yourself releasing these persons?

Visualize yourself with the courage and wisdom to let go of all those things which are no longer important or necessary in your life. Now look at the empty space you have cleared and create a landscape in a way that gives you joy and peacefulness. Now return to your breathing for a few more moments and then open your eyes and return to the present moment. Has this fantasy given you any ideas with which you want to follow through? How do you feel now about personal downsizing?

LOVE AND MARRIAGE
IN LATER MATURITY

The first 37 years were the hardest.
    --Suzanne Braun Levine, PBS Interview, LifePart2

Remember, sustaining a pleasurable, long-term marriage takes effort, deliberateness and an intention to learn about one another. In other words, marriage is for grown-ups
    --Cokie Roberts, From This Day Forward

I left my wife on a Monday night. My friend pulled his VW van up in front of the tiny, Spanish style house we were living in at the time, and we just started loading my things. I can still remember those two somber faces—my four-year-old son and my wife, thirty years his senior— as they sat on the couch and watched us go in and out of the house. Oh, I didn't take much in the way of material things, my clothes and my stereo, but what I took were pieces of our hearts. I hurt my wife a lot that night. Perhaps not more than she had hurt me over fifteen years of marriage, but who is to say who did what to whom, or who hurts the most in a failed marriage. My son was a little too young to understand all that was happening or what it was to mean for him, so he just sat in his mom's lap and watched my passage without a word. They both sat and stared in silence, and I guess I'll never forget those stares or the pain of that evening.

Leaving is always hard. Harder still if it means leaving those you really care about. I was so angry and so determined that night that I couldn't allow myself to consider their feelings. It had taken me an agonizingly long time to make the decision, and I wasn't stopping to reconsider. That night changed three lives forever. I wish I could tell you it was for the best, but after 33 years, I still don't honestly know. Some men—and some women as well— never look back when they leave their spouses and children, but I must confess that I have looked back a thousand times without an answer. Every moment of joy since that day has been tinged with the guilt and sadness that my son's life was never as secure and, perhaps, as fulfilling as it could have been if I had stayed. Every time my son went with his mother, I silently cursed myself for putting him in the position of having to adjust to life in two homes, and with two families. Every scene of a family having fun together, laughing and playing and just enjoying each other, left me empty and ashamed. Because I'm the one who decided to leave, I chose to carry this guilt squarely on my shoulders, and it has been a very heavy weight. I know that it is not healthy to feel guilt for this long, and would tell my clients the same, but like you, I'm still a work in progress.

What made me so unhappy that I had to leave? Why was I so dissatisfied? Was it me or was it her? I can think of many ways to answer these questions, but none of which assuage my guilt. I know now that I was asking my wife to be something she was not capable of being. I wanted her to love me freely and without reservation, but am now aware of how impossible that must have felt to her. I hoped she would be happy to see me when I got home and eager to find time to bring the baby and have lunch with me, but this disrupted a schedule she felt she had to adhere to. I wanted her to plan for fun times and commit to working through the difficult times, but planning, and committing, and working through our issues, was not something she felt capable of doing then. I yearned to have other children and enjoy raising them together, but she did not share this goal. These were the things I wanted and needed from my marriage, grew to believe they would never happen, and so made the decision to leave. I'm sure that if you asked her you would get similar responses of unmet needs and unfulfilled dreams.

It took me some time, but I did recover from the devastation of separation and divorce, and set about to start my life over at forty. With the help and encouragement of friends, I met some women, got onto a dating website, and started, tentatively, building new relationships. Most of these lasted less than a year. Eventually, I had a long-term relationship which, unfortunately, did not end with my goal of remarriage. I had mixed feelings about getting married again; both desiring to have another partner and worrying about how this would affect my son. He was always my priority, taking much of my time and attention, and as the years passed the window of opportunity to remarry began to close. I discovered that many of the women I met did not want to get married again. Although I am currently in a stable and fulfilling relationship, I remain single by choice—hers. I have learned a lot about myself and about intimate relationships in the past 33 years; one, specifically, is that love and sex can be just as wonderful as they were when you were young. There are some differences to be sure, mostly in the physical arena, but the ability to give and receive love can be enhanced by experience, seasoning, and maturity.

Although romantic love can be experienced just as fully in later maturity as in younger years, does this apply equally to marriage? Can the commitment of marriage to one person remain exciting and vibrant through the years, or does it inevitably fade over time? My editor, who's been married almost 25 years, thinks it can. She recently told me that she feels the same rush of excitement when she sees her husband after a day or two away, that she felt on their first date. "It all comes down to picking the right person," she says, "and not having unrealistic expectations." What are realistic expectations?

In a therapy session, a few months before my retirement, a young married woman exclaimed through her tears that "*you wouldn't hurt someone if you loved them.*" After a period of silence, I asked her to consider another point of view; that if you loved a person, were you not more willing to forgive them when they hurt you? We both looked at the possibility that if you wanted to be married for a long time, or for all time, it would be very important to learn how to forgive and how to ask for forgiveness. And that conversation made me think more about the thirty-seven years as a marriage therapist and all the boomer couples I've counseled along the way (you do a lot of reflection as you are about to retire). Are boomer marriages better or worse off than those of other generations? Are the divorce rates still as high for boomers today as they were during the late sixties, when they got so much publicity, or have the years helped the boomers see marriage in a different light and find the value of maintaining a long-term commitment?

I recently had the opportunity to talk with a former client about her 31-year marriage. Both Joan and her husband are boomers who have created a happy marriage through mutual effort and shared goals.

She stated that honesty, integrity, communication, and trust were the keys to their success. They have a swing on their porch that is designated as the place to talk about their relationship, and frequent conversations keep resentments from building. They were a little older than the norm when they got married and so they both had a chance to develop lives of their own. Now they can do things apart without it being a source of conflict. Because they are both self-motivated, there is not a lot of arguing about "who does what." But, above all else, she credits her husband for keeping them together, saying that "I would have left on many occasions if Ed had not been the one to give in and make changes for me."

Joan's evaluation of her marriage parallels the results of a 2014 study at the University of Rutgers. The researchers analyzed data collected from 394 couples, of which at least one member was 60 or older, and their average length of marriage was 39 years. Their findings indicate that the old maxim, "happy wife, happy life" remains true. The study showed that the more content the wife was in their relationship, the happier the husband felt, and this was despite his feelings about the relationship.

Further, the participants on average rated their general life satisfaction high (5 on a scale of 6), establishing a definite correlation between a highly-rated marriage and quality of life. The quality of marriage was shown to be very important in providing a "buffer" against the inevitable stressors and health issues of time and age (Carr & Freeman, 2014).

Commenting on the changes in women of this generation and their doubts about staying in long-term marriages, Suzanne Braun Levine writes, "Does a new lease on life mean having to walk away from a marriage of twenty or thirty years? Sometimes it does. Some women choose to leave—to escape constant conflict, deficient affection, emotional or physical abuse, simple emptiness. But for others of us, making changes in our lives can energize and transform marriages that we can no longer live within, but don't want to live without."[1]

There is no clear statistic as to how many boomers stayed in long-term marriages. There are statistics on the number of boomers who've married and subsequently divorced. The Fertility and Family Branch of the U.S. Census Bureau used this criterion in a 2001 survey and determined that the highest rate of divorce in any age group was 41 percent of men between 50 and 59, and 39 percent for women in the same age group. Well over half of boomer couples decided to stay in their first marriage. Although it is impossible to know if these marriages were happy or satisfying to each of the spouses, it can be said that a larger proportion of boomer couples honored their commitment to the institution of marriage at time when such a commitment was being seriously challenged.

To get some perspective on the failure of love and marriage for the boomers, we need to go back a few years and examine the particular history of our generation. It's been over 45 years since Woodstock, that hippie/boomer celebration of music, protest, and rebellion against established authority, beliefs, and societal norms. Boomers were just entering their twenties, with the oldest of them being twenty-three or twenty-four, and were shocking the country with their anti-establishment views and behaviors. With reckless abandon and total disrespect for the restrictive social conventions of their parents, they advocated "free love," protest marches, and the use of all kinds of illegal drugs, sometimes all during the same weekend. They supported civil rights, were anti-war, and, most importantly, the women's movement, openly attacking traditional gender roles and the institution of monogamous marriage. We boomers not only questioned what made a marriage successful or even tolerable, but whether marriage was viable in a time of social upheaval.

The divorce rate skyrocketed in the '70s, as the "leading edge" of the boomer generation began to leave their partners in large numbers in search of their own self-fulfillment. Many were fueled by the promise of free love and sexual explorations not possible in marriage. Second wave feminists regarded marriage as one more instrument of patriarchal oppression, and set out after a new kind of freedom. The institution of marriage was on the way to becoming at its best, optional, and at its worst, yesterday's news. As Pepper Schwartz, the love and relationship ambassador for AARP, and professor of sociology at the University of Washington recently wrote, "In many ways, divorce rates are the boomers' legacy."[2] This seems a sad legacy for the largest generation in U.S. history (somewhere in the neighborhood of 79 million) who believed so much in the promise of love.

We might assume that this is all history given that the Census Bureau reported that in the 1980s the divorce rate had started to flatten out and then decline. The numbers were wrong. When the American Community Survey came out in 2010, it became evident that the Census Bureau has been terribly shortsighted in its collection of divorce data over the last three decades. The data now indicates that the divorce rate for boomers, who are now 50 and older, doubled between 1990 and 2010. Over 600,000 boomers got divorced in 2010. Boomers were no more likely to get it right the second time: the rate of divorce for those in second marriages was 2.5 times as high as those in first marriages. The numbers of people ever divorced, currently divorced, or married at least twice are highest among those aged 50 and older, and one in three baby boomers is unmarried today—most of whom are either divorced or never-married, with only 10% widowed (Brown & Lin, 2012).

What this means is that our generation, which accounted for unprecedented divorce statistics through our youth, continues to lead the nation in unstable marriage and divorce. Apparently, we continue to search for a form of happiness that our marriages are not providing.

We were all having so much fun making love and not war: what happened when that notion of love came smack up against the realities of marriage? Researchers suggest many possible reasons for late-life divorce. Some categorize boomers as being narcissistic, incapable of making the compromises and self-sacrifices that contributed to the longevity of earlier generations' marriages. In this view, boomers define themselves as individuals first who show limited regard for the impact of their actions on their families. When a marriage feels empty and personally unfulfilling, boomers seem to find it easier to walk away than to stay and try to work things out—or perhaps our ancestors just suffered silently for the sake of propriety. Perhaps they had fewer idealistic illusions about marriage, or preferred staying married to the stigma of divorce. Indeed, the boomers as a generation see less shame in divorce. If a couple has grown apart, why shouldn't the individuals look to divorce as the best solution?

Other researchers look at the changes in the society in which the boomers grew up, citing the fact that women began to have more economic autonomy and could support themselves without being married. They no longer had to stay in unhappy or abusive marriages just to survive or ensure that their children were cared for. At the same time lay-offs and downsizing had left many men unemployed, underemployed, or hating the jobs that they had, leading to a general life dissatisfaction that was apt to leak into their perception of their marriages. When you look at the interaction between the changing economics of the times and the social upheavals of the 60s and 70s, it's not too hard to see why the institution of marriage became less important to boomers than it was for our parents.

Societal pressures played a significant role in my own divorce. So many of my peers were questioning the value of their marriages and then deciding to leave their spouses, that getting divorced almost felt like a rite of passage. Far too many of us supported one another in initiating divorce rather than asking for help, and few if any of my peers had extended family to which they could turn for advice. However, I cannot put the blame on outside pressures, for my divorce was a failure on both of our parts to look beyond our own needs and fears and understand that accepting your partner and giving freely without demanding something in return is the way to a successful and fulfilling marriage. It took me many years to learn that there is no specific way to happiness, you must find it in yourself.

So here we are, many of us divorced or remarried, single by choice or circumstance. Have we given up on love or are we still seeking it? Do we have realistic standards or are we still holding onto idealized notions of what it means to be in love or married?

Research and interviews with men and women of the boomer generation indicate that of the leading edge of this generation, women fared much better than men. At that time, divorce seemed a springboard for many women who were discovering their identities, while men felt a sense of failure and were often reluctant to return to single life. But as the second wave of boomers, referred to as "Jonesers," began to experience divorce, the differences in the sexes in terms of how they adjusted, also began to change. The American Community Survey (ACS), conducted in 2010, indicated that 30% of middle-aged and older adults were in remarriages, although the odds of divorce were roughly 40% higher than for those in first marriages. Further research of unmarried boomers highlighted their vulnerability as compared with married boomers: they were disproportionately younger, non-white women, who tended to have fewer economic resources and poorer health, and to live alone (Lin & Brown, 2012). As both the leading edge of the boomer generation and the Jonesers grow older, they will face some significant issues.

The secret to a better adjustment following the shock of divorce seemed to be the amount of social support rather than financial status (this excludes those who were left in virtual poverty). Women, both during marriage and after divorce, placed a much greater value on their friendships with other women, while divorced men had few friends and were less likely to have the support of their children. Many men, however, finding that the ratio of unmarried women to men was in their favor, set out to find new partners. Dating websites began to flourish and it was much easier to get a date or get into a serious relationship. This was a major factor in the significant increase in remarriages for those in later maturity. Though boomer marriages often ended with bitterness and recrimination, many survivors of these failed marriages resumed their search for happiness. Deirdre Bair in her book, *Calling It Quits*, reports that "The word they all use, in one form or another is 'happiness.' They speak of the 'quest' for it, the 'pursuit' of it, the 'desire' for it, and usually a statement like this one follows: 'I am entitled to have it."[3]

The strength of that pursuit has led to changes in the relationships themselves. Although "living alone together" (referred to as LAT by the statisticians) has been part of the life style of the very wealthy, it has now become an acceptable option for those of lesser means. As a regular demographic category, it refers to those couples in a committed relationship who choose to maintain separate residences and only stay together by agreement. The LAT, is another statistic that can be added to the boomer legacy.

One positive finding that can be teased out of all the statistics on boomer divorce is that 70% of those who remain married are in first marriages, and that once these couples get beyond the 18 to 20-year mark, they generally remain married for the rest of their lives. These marriages are not without problems, but it is the couples' commitment to each other and to their marriage, that sustains them through rough times. As Laura revealed in our interview, it was her husband who made the necessary changes to keep their marriage together. It seems incumbent upon men to learn more satisfying and effective marital skills, and for women to let go of their unrealistic standards. In a PBS special called LifePart2, Terrence Real, marital therapist and author of the book, *The New Rules of Marriage*, said this about the boomers' quest for love and fulfillment:

"I believe that both sexes, but particularly women vocally, are saying, I want this marriage to be a marriage I want to be in, not one I need to be in. I think we really want to be lifelong lovers. We want to have great sex, 20, 30 years into our marriages, we want to be emotionally connected and intimate. I don't think what people really get is that these are brand-new demands on marriage. We want the same things that you would have gotten in an early-stage relationship, in an affair, in a novel. And we want it for the rest of our lives."[4]

Real goes on to say that men have responded to these new demands by calling them unrealistic and expecting their wives to accept less. He suggests that this isn't a solution but that women are going to have to be empowered in a way that both helps themselves and helps men rise to the occasion. This will take relationship skills up to the level of our new ambition, and as he mentions, no one teaches girls or boys these types of relationship skills.

My work with couples over the years has led me to agree with Real's assessment that the institution of marriage has been in crisis for the past 50 years. I met with men running from the women they saw as overly demanding and incapable of compromise. I met with women unburdening themselves of men they perceived as controlling and abusive, as they refused to be victimized anymore. But, there were fewer couples with whom I met who were willing to do the hard work of trying to understand the other, working through their resentments, facing their fears, and taking responsibility for their own failures in the relationship. These are major factors in the escalating divorce rate among middle-aged and older adults.

Further, I think that men need to learn how to support one another in finding a new model of strength—based on personal responsibility, compassion, and cooperation—that we can bring to our marriages and committed new relationships. In conjunction with those changes, I think that women need to reclaim the softness devalued over the past half century, and change their idealized expectations and demands into a loving form of guidance, both for their men and for their children. The Women's Movement is incomplete if it doesn't come full circle and work together with men in creating a new paradigm for love relationships, whether within the institution of marriage or other types of partnerships. I would like to suggest this as a new boomer legacy.

For the men and women who courageously campaigned and fought for same-sex marriage, I applaud and support your efforts. While it is beyond the scope of this book to go into detail, it is extremely important to recognize your accomplishments. Many in our country vehemently oppose this movement toward equality, but I feel that the risks that have been taken for the sake of love and commitment may be just what the rest of us need to re-examine our own willingness to stand up for what we believe. Perhaps boomers of all sexual orientations can come together in solidarity to give new life to the institution of marriage.

So here we are: the youngest of us in our 50s and the oldest starting our 70s, and many of us still want to have more fulfilling relationships with our existing partners or to get married again. What are the qualities that can make marriage remain vital and exciting through the years? As a marriage therapist for so many years I've seen many bad marriages and a few good ones, but certainly none that were perfect. The reality is: if you want to have the relationship of your dreams, you have to work at it. To this end I am going to present some ideas adapted to the specific needs of couples in later maturity. I will try to stay away from the advice of the Beatles that "all you need is love," as well as the "10 things that will make marriage better" lists that populate the internet these days.

My first and most important piece of advice is: **WHEN YOU DON'T NEED IT, IT WILL COME TO YOU!** Think about this for a minute. Try to understand that whenever we try to coerce or manipulate our partners to provide what we need— validation, comfort, sex, compliments—we always get resistance, and this in turn leads to anger and hurt feelings, and statements like "you never.. ." or "if you loved me. . ." Learn to take care of your own needs first and what you want from the other person will be more likely to come to you without asking. One of my clients credits this principle with saving his marriage. All his efforts were in trying to get his wife to behave in ways that met his needs. When he began to focus on meeting his own needs and not being dependent upon her, the intense pressure that had developed between them was reduced and she felt that she could give him what he wanted by choice and not by coercion.

The boomer generation rebelled against the tyranny of the marital patterns they saw in their parents. Now it's time to practice the skills that our parents did not have. When this husband took responsibility for his own needs, his wife saw him as much more attractive as well. Marriage is no longer two people becoming one in mutual dependence. That's the old model. Marriage can now be between two independent people who choose to come together out of love and mutual respect. Fortunately, I was able to help this client work through issues from his past so that he could present to his wife a more mature, more independent version of the man she had married. That is why some of my best marital therapy was done individually.

Stop trying to convince your partner of your point of view and start learning how to tolerate and/or understand theirs. Spouses don't have to agree on everything or see everything the same way. My experience with boomer couples is that many of their disagreements turn into an argument over "who's right and who's wrong." From my perspective, boomer marriages have become more of a power struggle than the marriages I saw earlier in my career. Unfortunately, there is no resolution for the right/wrong argument, because *we all feel that we are right and our partner is wrong*. With this mindset, communication amounts to waiting, impatiently at best, for our partner to finish speaking, so we can state our side of things one more time. Listening to one another and trying to understand what your spouse is really saying has somehow been lost. Women are speaking up in powerful ways now, and so listening skills are even more important than before; when a man could dominate a conversation or, on the other hand, hide behind the paper. Finding statements that communicate you are listening to your partner and are interested in what he or she is saying, clarifying when you don't understand, and staying calm when you respond, are skills that we all can improve on. Years ago, a man said to me, "What could a woman possibly say that could interest me." I knew that man was in deep trouble. That attitude, from either a man or a woman, cannot fly in today's marital climate.

The rules of fair fighting apply to all couples everywhere. These are rules for communication during an argument or conflict. Basically, they implore us to avoid name calling and other aggressive behaviors, to be specific and stick to the matter at hand, not bringing up other issues or old battles. They advise us to stop pointing the finger at the other person in generalizations that are apt to cause defensiveness, such as "you never" or "you always," and instead to simply state what you want or need. They demand that we stop interrupting our partners, and call a time out when things get too heated. I always advise couples to take a walk or do something different for a brief period of time. But always, always, come back and finish the discussion in a more peaceful way.

Don't leave the quality of your marriage to chance, because if you do you may just recreate the marriage of your parents. If you do not feel like going to a marriage counselor, then read books and articles about successful marriage.

Learn to work as a team, having open communication about important mutual issues, such as money, in-laws, your adult children, grandchildren, and so on. There are more outside pressures on marriage than ever before, especially when both spouses work. Family schedules can become overwhelming and a potential source of resentment. What one partner perceives as an unfair division of the workload is a frequent cause of stress. With the current demands on our time, it is important to have a mutual agreement as to who does what, when, and how often, and a clearly designated time and place for weekly communication over this and other ongoing issues. Even more than that, though, is the need to share your deepest feelings, hopes and dreams about your marriage and about life in general. This is what builds real intimacy.

Work toward a delicate balance between being close and allowing one another space. Today's couples, especially those in later maturity, have more independence for their own interests, sometimes even going on separate trips and vacations. The time apart and then reuniting can bring renewed vitality.

Make affection and sex a priority. I advise couples to have a weekly or at least bi-monthly date night. Some of us in later maturity just allow our sex lives to diminish, and with it the expression of affection as well. Earlier generations may have just accepted that marriages become sexless with the passage of time, but as boomers, we can do something about this. With the advancement of medications for ED, and the use of hormone replacement therapy, couples can expect to be sexually active into their later years. This can be both a blessing and a curse, as spouses may have differing desires or physical limitations. Being creative and resourceful in keeping a sex life active and enjoyable may require the assistance of a physician or a therapist. It also may require an agreement to remain affectionate but not engage in sexual activity. It is vitally important to have intimate conversations about our sexual relationships, so that a loving solution can be reached.

Take responsibility for your own feelings and quit blaming your partner. If you want a healthy relationship, be the first to admit your part in an argument or disagreement, and see what happens.

Try to follow the advice of Don Miguel Ruiz and "never make assumptions." I experienced this so much in my work with couples. Something would happen that was annoying and one or both would interpret their partner's motive, often in the worst possible light, never checking it out with them, believing their own judgments, and then feeling justified in becoming hurt and angry. In our session, they would be shocked to find that the way they saw the situation was a projection of their own beliefs and judgments. By then these assumptions may have led to a huge argument. Sometimes words were said that could not be taken back. Learn to check things out first. "Motives like stowaways," wrote W.H. Auden, "are found too late," and this is sadly true in marriage.

Accept your partner for who he or she is, not who you might want them to be, for this is not love. Love is accepting and kind, looking for the positive and not nit-picking the negative. Work toward becoming your partner's biggest cheer leader, supporting their personal growth and care for their health. This also means not trying to fix your partner. I used to see this mostly in men who are hard wired to fix things, but now I see it in both sexes. Acceptance and support go a long way toward a happy marriage.

Be aware that you do not have a God given right to comment or pass judgment on everything your partner says or does. Learn when to remain silent and just listen for a change: you may find that your partner is very appreciative. If you really want to take a risk, ask them to tell you more, to clarify anything you didn't understand, and even remark about your interest in their thoughts and actions. If you are truly interested in your partner, it will be reciprocated.

What about dating in later maturity? What are realistic expectations? With approximately 26 million single boomers, and internet dating sites that enable us to check out potential partners around the world, dating after age 50 is a real possibility. Having been married for fifteen years, and single for the past thirty-one, I've developed some perspective on the subject. Although I still believe that marriage is the best option for the future of humanity, if I had to choose which was more interesting in terms of both love and growth potential, I would have to say the latter. The reasons I draw this conclusion are as follows:

Dating can be more fun when you are on equal footing with the opposite sex. There is not as much to prove in later maturity and not as much at stake with every date. Some dates work out, some do not, but getting to know someone, even if just over a cup of coffee, can only help to improve your social skills. The balance of power in marriage is a little more unstable in my opinion, and requires more work to keep its equilibrium. Equal footing is a little easier to accomplish when both parties are putting their best foot forward.

Courting can bring a new sense of exhilaration and keep you young. Many boomers complain that it's "too much like work" to establish a new relationship, but I think it is just a matter of choice.

There is much more emphasis on getting to know a potential partner as a person first. Studies have shown that a friendship is always the best basis for a lasting relationship. With new information about relationships in general, and with an awareness of what did not work in the past, dating can be a time to get to know a person in more depth before making a commitment. However, recent evidence shows that second marriages are more prone to divorce than first marriages, so apparently, not enough single boomers are using this time wisely.

Learning dating skills at a later age can make up for many of the feelings of inadequacy we all experienced earlier in our lives. Like many of you, I was intimidated by the opposite sex and the whole process of dating. If not for the church, I wouldn't have had any girlfriends in high school or college. The church provided a more comfortable environment for meeting and getting to know the opposite sex. Now you can improve your dating skills with the help and advice of dating coaches, much as you might have seen in the movie *Hitch*.

Sex can be wonderfully fulfilling when you can take your time, explore new possibilities, and not take it so seriously. Of course, this is just as applicable to marriage, but single life provides opportunities to learn from different partners the art of timing and playfulness that can enhance the sexual experience. It also creates more interest and motivation to keep romance alive. My work with both single people and married couples—as well as my own experience—underscores that those in a dating relationship find sex more exciting when they know they will only see their partner for one or two nights a week, whereas married couples complain that their sex life is boring or they don't have sex as often as when they were dating or newly married. However, each single person must decide what is morally and ethically acceptable for his or her sense of self-worth and integrity. Risk and reward are both high in this area of single life. Practicing safe sex, being faithful within a relationship, and never using anyone for your own sexual gratification are good rules to follow.

New "sexual enhancements" make it possible to have a sexual relationship much later in life. Boomers can utilize a variety of prescription drugs and natural supplements, lotions and toys, to have sex into their eighties—or maybe longer. Who knows what advances in this area are on the horizon? I can imagine that we will eventually have an "app" you can download to your phone which will guarantee better sex.

Later maturity can be a time to experience love and sex free from the fears that held us back before, or, if one is open, to work through old fears and wounds, and love more fully and unreservedly. You no longer need to find a soul mate, just a mate who has a soul. If you have been single for as many years as I have, you know that there is no one who is perfect for you, so you need to give up idealistic expectations or be constantly disappointed. Being single forces you to learn the art of bargaining and compromise, sometimes in working out the details of a first date.

I once called a woman that I had met online, to meet me for the first time. During that conversation, a conflict came up that irritated me so much I said: "let's forget the whole thing." She immediately changed her argumentative stance and then began pursuing me for a place and time to meet. I would have never been so bold before, but being single has taught me a few things, especially how to keep good boundaries.

We finally settled on a mutually acceptable time and place, and had an enjoyable time together. After our initial greeting, she told me that she had plans to meet her girlfriend later, and I agreed that this was fine with me. She later excused herself to "phone her girlfriend and cancel." We talked and got to know each other, but this was one of those dates that did not lead to any further dating. What I learned was that I had the right to speak my truth, even if it was negative, and not be afraid of the outcome.

You can have separate beds and separate residences without all the guilt. You too can become a "living alone together." When the morning comes and you must go to work or want to do something by yourself, it's nice to know that your relationship partner is equally happy to be on their own. Texting then becomes a technological miracle, keeping you connected through the week when you don't have the time for a phone conversation. As mature adults, however, I hope that we all continue to use a phone for the purpose it was intended—to speak to another human being.

You don't have to be quiet because of the kids. In fact, you don't have to be quiet at all. So many boomers are living alone now, with their children raised and on their own, making it possible to experience the privacy to focus on one another without distractions.

When you feel too tired to go looking for someone, you can just go to your computer to see who is available in the area of your choice. You might even enjoy learning the subtleties of online dating. I know that I felt challenged by what to write, and how to phrase what I really wanted to say. By trial and error I eventually found the right things to say to attract a woman, and this became a source of pride and a sense of accomplishment. Every once and a while my girlfriend wistfully mentions the fun we had writing back and forth. When I am inspired, I send her emails as if we were still in that early stage of getting to know one another, keeping the romance in our relationship.

You now feel infinitely more grateful for a good date, for good conversation, and if that date leads to sex, for a good orgasm. It is not nearly as easy to take things for granted. For many of us, this provides the opportunity and the impetus for self-improvement. Self-help books aren't just for women, you know. I challenge both sexes to make single living and dating a time for personal growth as a relationship partner, and as human beings living in this particular time of history. Loving and being loved is one of the most profound experiences of life. It deserves our complete attention and commitment.

One last personal note: the writing of this book and especially this chapter has caused me to revisit many events in my past, and not without considerable grief. During this time, I have worked very hard to try to resolve some left-over issues with my ex-wife regarding our divorce. Through email, we communicated back and forth. Some of my emails were well received while others caused disagreements and periods during which she withdrew from contact with me. Feeling that this was very important to me, to my ex-wife, and ultimately to our son, I continued to reach out to her, apologizing for whatever wrongs I had done, even after all this time. I shared with her those events that were the most painful for me, hoping she would understand. Allowing a vulnerability I hadn't seen since we were together, she apologized and took responsibility for her inner process during that time in her life. I found her words tremendously healing, and can honestly say that after more than thirty years, I feel we have finally forgiven each other. Along with her apology she shared with me the following poem, written as part of her own healing process:

I was 18. You were 23.
So very young, carrying childhood
wounds we each thought the other
could heal somehow.
All we ever wanted in our heart of
hearts was to love and be loved.
That is the heartache buried so
many years ago under layers of
anger and fear, like concrete poured
over our dreams of romance, fun, and
the family life we each seemed to long
for since the beginning of time.
How could we have known? No one ever
taught us that all we had to do was leave
the past behind, and sing our Soul Songs
together like two Morning Doves greeting
each other in the new day sun
It never had to be so hard,
but how could we have known?

Bonnie Joyce Walker

I said earlier that these years would bring new challenges as well as new opportunities, and we might all need to embrace change as a way of life. Nowhere is this truer than in the area of love and relationships. For those who are married the challenge is keeping love alive and vital through the passage of time. For those who are single comes the opportunity of meeting someone who makes your heart beat just a little faster once more. The excitement lies in the choices we all have. "Grow old along with me," penned Robert Browning, "the best is yet to be. . ."

Do you have the courage to make this a reality?

EXERCISE #7

FACE TRACING FOR COUPLES

This exercise focuses on becoming more aware of your partner without the use of words, as we work on tracing one another's face. Although any couple could benefit from going through the following steps, I found that many of the boomer couples I worked with had become so accustomed to their partner that they no longer looked at each other with the intimacy that I am suggesting in this exercise. Sometimes we forget to genuinely look at our partner to see the unspoken things that are revealed in the language of their face. Try to stay focused and open as you proceed through the following steps and see what happens.

Sit in two comfortable chairs facing each other. Just take a moment to relax as you look into each other's eyes. Decide which one of you will go first. One of you should close your eyes and sit as still as possible. The other should look into your partner's face and become aware of all its features and details. Remember, this is a nonverbal exercise, so, without talking, and without touching your partner's face, begin to move your finger over his or her features as if you were drawing a sketch. . . As you do this, notice which side of the face seems dominant and which less dominant. Continue this sketching motion on the less dominant side. Now make contact and begin to stroke this side of your partner's face very lightly as your fingers move. Imagine that the touch of your fingers draws out these features and brings them to life. Now slowly withdraw your hand and give your partner some time to absorb the experience.

Now switch roles, and without talking, repeat the exercise. First, look closely at your partner's face, and then draw your partner's features with your finger without touching them. Then notice which side of the face seems less dominant and begin to touch this less dominant side of the face gently. Now, draw out these features and try bringing them to life. Then slowly withdraw your hand and give your partner some time to absorb his or her experience.[1]

Take the next 5 to 10 minutes (or longer if you need) to talk with your partner about, but not limited to the following:

1. What did you experience during the face tracing?

2. What did you see when you really looked at your partner? Were you able to see the life experience in your partner's face? What do the changes in your partner's face say about your relationship?

3. If your relationship is fairly new, what did you learn about your partner that has been unspoken before?

4. What did you see in one side that made it seem less dominant?

5. How did it feel to have that side drawn out? Did it feel supportive or scary?

6. What did you feel toward your partner during the exercise?

7. One side of this exercise requires intense focus, while the other side requires a bit of surrender. How can you use these skills to improve your relationship?

In workshops that I have led this exercise always elicits a lot of emotion and more than a few tears. The de-briefing afterward is generally spirited and often leads to new insights about the relationship and sometimes about each person who participates. One person had an injury to the "less dominant" side of her face when she was very young and had never spoken about it until we did the exercise. She openly expressed her pain and later reported being very grateful for the experience.

I hope you find this exercise as insightful as others have reported.

STRATEGIES FOR SINGLES

Many boomers find themselves single again after years of being married, whether due to death or divorce, and now face the prospect of trying to find companionship in a very scary and uncertain dating scene. At this point many people just give up, saying it's too hard to meet someone, too emotionally hazardous to go on dates, or that they just don't have the will or the energy to work on a new relationship. I have heard all of these excuses. It is difficult. It can be painful or just a hassle to start a new relationship. I cannot tell you how many times I picked up the phone to ask a woman for a date and put it down again and again because I could not muster the courage or the emotional energy.

What happens is that your brain, in a supreme effort to protect you from hurt, humiliation, or failure, sets up a number of roadblocks to stop you from trying. An inner voice whispers, "What are you going to say, anyway?" Another voice regales you with, "This is just too much stress." And if that isn't enough, your memory center flashes pictures of every failure you've had with the opposite sex. You're exhausted and you haven't even started the process. Better to put down the phone or shut down your email and have some ice cream.

While you have to admire your brain for its attempt to keep you from some imaginary form of emotional pain, this is actually backwards thinking. What needs to happen is for you to get the tenacity to overcome your roadblocks and fears, and start controlling your thoughts rather than being controlled by them. And ultimately, that is all they are—thoughts. They do not define you any more than a freckle on your chin does. You are more than your thoughts. Come on man, get some fortitude. Come on woman, show some guts. If you are going to be successful at single life, you must learn to get out of your comfort zone and take some risks.

Getting Started:

1. Make a list of all your fears concerning the possibility of meeting someone new and/or dating.

2. Take the list to your shredder and shred it.

3. Rewrite the list changing the fears into

challenges. If you wrote, "I'm afraid of meeting someone new," now write something like, "I look forward to meeting someone new." If you wrote "I'm afraid of being rejected," now write something like, "I have the courage to face rejection.

4. Go to your computer and google "singles activities in my area," or "singles activities for 50+."

5. Get on a dating site. You can start with some of the free ones to get a feel for what works for you.

6. Do not put your entire history on your profile, just enough to make you interesting. Leave a little mystery to create some intrigue.

7. Develop a style of responding to potential matches that sets you apart. I used to start a limerick and ask potential dates to complete it. Comment positively on his or her profile photograph, and keep it simple and light hearted. Don't resort to clichés—I always

hated it when someone talked about drinking wine and having long walks on the beach—blah, blah, blah. Don't be afraid to reveal something more personal and specific to you. Even mentioning a specific beach that you like is preferable to a cliché.

8. When you meet for the first time, make it a public place for coffee or tea. If you don't like the person you just met, you have only invested a little time, and have done so in a place where you each have an easy exit strategy if need be.

9. Always have a backup plan, that is, something you tell your date that you have to do later, like meet up with some friends, etc.

10. This is supposed to be fun, so enjoy yourself.

11. One date is not a life time commitment.

12. Remember, when a little voice inside your head says, "yep, he's just like my ex-husband," or "she could never replace my former wife," these are only thoughts that have little to do with the other person. It's

really a smokescreen that you brain creates to keep you from taking any chances. Just let those thoughts drift out of your head and return to enjoying the moment. Who knows, sitting across from you could be the chance of a lifetime.

13. If you are hitting it off and it seems like there might be something there, suggest a second date, but make it simple and non-threatening.

14. If it turns into a dating relationship, take it slow and keep your options open.

15. Know what you want in a partner, and don't settle for less.

With all this being said, being single in the second half of life can be filled with excitement or dread. It's what you make of it that's important.

**Note: If you find yourself having the same negative thoughts or repeating the same negative patterns that cause new relationships to fall apart, it's time to seek professional help.

WHO IS IN YOUR CIRCLE?

No man is an island. . .every man is a piece of a continent, a part of the main.

--John Donne Meditation XVII

In the years since Donne penned those words, a tremendous amount of research has been done on the human brain, much of it supporting the legendary poet in the conclusion that the brain is a social organ, and that human beings were not meant to live alone. This is vitally important in childhood and equally meaningful throughout the aging process as well. It has been well documented that the need to belong is basic to human existence. Abraham Maslow made it one of the basic building blocks in his hierarchy of needs, while current research focuses on the desire for interpersonal attachment as fundamental to human motivation. Belonging is more than attachment, however, for it brings with it the opportunity to be more than oneself, to be part of a much larger community—humanity itself.

If the need to belong, to be connected to other human beings in a significant way is so important, why are so many aging Americans isolated, lonely, and alone? Often it is because friends and family move away or die, and many of us lack the physical energy to venture out and make new connections. Younger people seem to regard us as irrelevant, or worse—invisible. We don't see well enough to feel comfortable driving at night or we don't hear well, so find the ambient noise of restaurants or other places where people gather, annoying. Chronic health problems isolate us as we don't feel we'd make good company for anyone else, or perhaps our social engagements with our peers have become such whine-fests that we long for the company of younger, healthier people. Once we've confined ourselves to the comfort of our apartments or homes with only our TVs or computers for company, we become the victims of inertia. There are many reasons why we can become isolated as we age, but it is important to keep from letting loneliness overtake us.

Basically, loneliness is a disease. It creeps up on you when your resistance is down. Like sub-clinical cases of physical illnesses, it can lie dormant in your psyche for the better part of a lifetime just waiting for the right set of circumstances to become evident. Oh, there's the occasional isolated cough or solitary sniffle, or even the extended blues influenza to let you know that its dangers lurk in even the most innocuous life situations. Maybe it's part of the human experience, like sickness or aging itself. You can call these feelings disillusionment, loneliness or abandonment, but when it hits you, it can really lay you low.

Colleagues tell me that loneliness and being alone are two different things, that some people can be alone for extended periods of time and not experience loneliness at all. They "enjoy their own company" or are so immersed in creative work or hobbies that they don't need the distraction of other people. That's certainly not the case for me.

Being alone is ok for a time, but when it passes a certain threshold, it turns into bitter, gut wrenching loneliness; the feeling that everyone has abandoned you, leaving you without a place in the universe. One isolated woman reported her feelings of loneliness as coming "In waves, like a fever." Many of the people I have had the privilege of working with, talk a great deal about the anxiety they experience at the thought of being alone, and the ever-present feelings of doubt about their place in the world. They experience tremendous uncertainty about being accepted, about their worthiness to be loved. And that's what I think is at the heart of loneliness: the belief that we aren't loved after all. Maybe we can fool others for a time, or get by for a while on good performance, but one big slip-up, one major mistake, and we will be exposed for who we really are: stowaways on the ship of life. This, I believe, is what makes human beings feel lonely, and alone. It is the belief that if we aren't loved, then we stand alone in the universe without anyone to say that we counted, that our lives mattered.

Recent Census Bureau findings indicate that more than one in four households are occupied by just one person. To highlight the substantial increase, the ratio of one-person households in 1970 was one in six. Over 33 million Americans are now living alone.

Given the data that Americans are marrying later, having fewer children, divorcing at higher rates, and are living longer than before, it stands to reason that many in our country will find themselves living alone, either temporarily or permanently. The largest demographic of people living by themselves are boomers age and older, with about 10% of all households in this country being single people 65 and over. Although there is no accurate data separating the two, some live alone out of necessity, but many are making it a life style choice. As later maturity continues to evolve to a longer and more active time of life, boomers are choosing their independence and freedom to live as they please, regardless of the possibilities of loneliness and isolation.

Whether by choice or circumstance, living alone can be fraught with difficulties. This makes it even more important to cultivate and nurture a social circle of friends, family, and associates as we move through later maturity into retirement and old age. Many people leave relationships behind as they leave the workplace, or make a geographic move, often for financial reasons or to escape weather they can no longer tolerate. It's entirely too easy to become isolated as health, personal, family or financial problems make just getting through the day difficult. But the challenge for all of us is to work harder at keeping our current friends, deepening our relationships with family members, and taking the risk of making new friends. By most accounts, women seem to be better at creating and maintaining friends, so it is more urgent that men begin to practice their social skills; finding ways to get acquainted with somebody new or repair a friendship that has been diminished over time. For those who have lost touch with their families because of past issues or general family dysfunction, it may mean "adopting" people with whom you choose to create close familial ties. If you lack grandchildren, there are programs that assist you in becoming a grandparent to a needy child. A friend of mine volunteers as a reading coach in a local elementary school and loves it. Another friend has established a close relationship with a college student who helps him become more proficient with his computer. The computer work takes the first third of their time and the rest is spent in lively conversation. It's hard to say who is learning the most is this intergenerational relationship. AARP is also involved in getting out information about communities that have age-friendly programs aimed at reducing isolation by promoting the very same intergenerational networking and socialization. Finally, we all need to be open to utilizing the community services that assist with getting people our age together, like meet-up groups or senior centers. I know, you don't want to hang out with all those old people, but go down there and see what kind of activities are available before you make a judgment. I have taken several community classes for seniors and found them to be a lot of fun. One of those was a Windows 7 class that helped immensely with the writing of this book. Who Knew?

There are times, however, when a relationship has run its course and is now causing more stress to maintain than the joy it provides from getting together. Occasionally, the interests and values that have kept a friendship together change, leaving each person tense and anxious when thinking about spending time together. When this happens, it is much better to face the reality that this relationship no longer works, and it would be better for everybody to let it go. Later maturity is a time for evaluating all our relationships, and letting go of those that no longer meet our needs.

In the process of evaluation, however, those of us in later maturity need to examine whether we share some responsibility for the isolation and the resulting loneliness we feel, if, in fact, past offenses and injuries inflicted by parents, spouses, or friends can finally be resolved, old wounds forgiven and healed. Remaining hurt or angry over events that happened long in the past is a burden too many of us carry. Those burdens cause a whole host of physical and emotional consequences. They may lead us to avoid making new friendships, reinforcing our own growing isolation. None of us wants to become the stereotype of the bitter, cranky old person who drives other people away. Though many of us may feel shortchanged by life or entitled to our bitterness, these are reactions guaranteed to isolate us further.

Often people are reluctant to forgive past slights or even major violations because they question whether the victimizer deserves forgiveness after committing such acts as abuse, molestation, unfaithfulness, or even more unspeakable acts. Others fear that if they forgive their victimizer, they leave themselves open to a continuation of the same behavior. A client once said to me when I suggested she forgive her mother after years of working on her hurt and anger, "What, and let her off the hook?" She felt that I was encouraging something grossly unfair to her own sense of integrity. At the same time, she showed little awareness of how she was internalizing her resentment and anger and displacing it onto others. In her case, I felt that holding on to her long-standing resentment was also causing numerous physical problems. Once she worked on forgiving her mother and letting go of all the negative feelings, many of her physical symptoms disappeared.

The question that all of us should ask: does forgiveness help? All the research on forgiveness indicates that by letting go and pardoning the hurtful acts of others, we can lower our blood pressure and depressive symptoms, and probably reduce our risk of cardiovascular disease. There is evidence that post-traumatic symptoms are reduced, interpersonal relationships with those we forgive get better, and as people reach later maturity, they have better overall physical and mental health. Forgiveness, it seems, is good for us in many ways.[1]

There are two basic components to forgiveness: the initial letting go of the pain, anger, and need for revenge connected with the victimizer, and the possibility of restoring a relationship that has been damaged. Forgiveness is always a possibility while restoring a relationship is a more difficult task and sometimes impossible. The first part requires a person to validate the intensity of feelings, and then make a choice to let go of past pain, the need for revenge, and the constant focus on the injury itself. Setting strong boundaries for your own protection is essential if your wish is to try to restore the fractured relationship.[2]

For many people this is not possible, for parents have died, victimizers have disappeared or may even be incarcerated, and few people are willing to work through the steps that would complete the process of forgiveness. Although this is disappointing, it cannot prevent you from getting the closure you need through the symbolic acts outlined above.

Forgiving yourself for misunderstandings and misguided behaviors is extremely important to the closure you seek. So many of us, myself included, hold onto regrets and perceived failures because at an unconscious level we feel the need to be punished. An inner voice reminds us that we do not deserve good things in our life, because of past wrong doings. The years of rumination and self-recriminations may be equally, or even more damaging to our physical and emotional health than holding grudges against others. In this regard, forgiveness is a gift you give to yourself, not those who have injured you, for it allows you to return to present reality, gain valuable insight, and move on with your life. If you feel you need help, it would be wise to see a professional who can assist you with the process. Perhaps the following illustration will inspire you.

In the movie, The Railway Man, Colin Firth plays the part of Eric Lomax, a British soldier captured by the Japanese during the fall of Singapore in 1942. In this true story, based on his best-selling memoir, Lomax is forced to work on the notorious "death railway" from Thailand to Burma, during which time he is severely beaten, water boarded, and locked in a bamboo cage of about the size that would house a large dog. Despite the hardships, he survives to confront his tormentor 40 years later. As Rex Reed writes in his review, "It's an inspiring and unforgettable story about cruelty, endurance, courage and making peace with the past"[3]

The early scenes depict the meeting and marriage of Lomax and wife Patti, but also the severe symptoms of post-traumatic stress from which he suffers, and his obsession to seek revenge on the sadistic Japanese translator, Nagase. It was Nagase's treacherous interrogation of Lomax that was greatly responsible for much of his torture, and so he is the target of Lomax's hatred. Through another POW, he learns that his nemesis is still alive, and in fact, is leading tours through the old railroad internment camp.

Lomax decides he must confront Nagase and torture him in the ways in which he was tortured himself, and fantasizes about killing him. When they finally meet again, he reveals his identity and begins his own interrogation. In their heated exchanges, Nagase moves from denial and defensiveness, to being openly fearful. Finally, as Nagase begins to express his remorse, Lomax softens, opening the door for Nagase to surrender to his need for forgiveness. Though Lomax is not ready for total forgiveness, he feels compassion for this guilt-ridden man, and the process of healing begins for both men. As the movie ends, snapshots of them together in various locations, suggest that they eventually became friends.

This remarkable story of courage and healing reminds us that we always have a choice to change the way we think and feel. People who are aging successfully do whatever it takes to overcome past events and the subsequent life patterns that no longer suit their needs. They are committed to personal growth throughout the life cycle.

The question: who's in your circle? is one that all of us need to consider carefully. Building and maintaining a strong social support system, finding ways to be actively involved with others, or deciding to take the necessary steps to get out of the isolation that might be your current life situation, are all very important steps for successful aging. It remains an ever-present challenge for the boomer generation and for all of us in the second half of life.

EXERCISE #8

One wonderful way of brightening your spirits and strengthening the bonds of an important friendship is the Gratitude Visit. Here are the steps to follow:

Think of someone whom you should thank, someone who has been helpful or kind to you. Pick someone that you ought to thank more than you have.

1. Write a letter to that person. Make it a real tribute, a page of your thoughts and recollections. Tell the person how they helped you and how that affected you later in your life.

2. Writing the letter longhand is shown to have more positive effect than typing it on a computer.

3. Frame or laminate the letter.

4. Call your friend and ask for a time to come by

and visit. Tell your friend you have something to read to them. Then visit them, read your letter, and leave it with them.

I hope you will find this to be a very rewarding experience for both you and your friend.

*Adapted from: "The Healing Power of a Gratitude Visit" Copyright 2009 Lynn D. Johnson. Contact: Lynn Johnson, Ph.D., Tel: (801) 261-1412; E-mail: drj@enjoylifebook.com

RELIGION OR SPIRITUALITY?

Your hearts know in silence the secrets
Of the days and the nights.
But your ears thirst for the sound of
your heart's knowledge.

--Kahlil Gibran, *The Prophet*

Religion and spirituality are not the same thing. A person can be deeply spiritual, but not religious at all. Conversely, a person can be very religious and yet not exhibit many spiritual characteristics. This is because religion is generally recognized to be the organization of spiritual values into specific denominations, beliefs and practices, while spirituality encompasses a much broader set of internal beliefs about the nature of reality and our part in the larger universe. While religion focuses on following the teachings of a specific prophet or divine figure such as Yahweh, Jesus, Mohammed, or Buddha, spirituality is more of an open-ended view of the greater reality and the possibilities that exist for human interaction within that reality. Religion helps us establish our place in the world, while spirituality invites us to move beyond traditional beliefs and concepts and search for more.

The practice of religion gives people social support, security, and a sense of belonging through their specific religious affiliation. Research indicates that 40 to 60 percent of all religious congregations are composed of retired persons, and most older adults report that religion helps them cope with the inevitable losses and difficulties of aging. Other studies suggest that people who attend some type of religious service weekly extend their lives by as much as seven years. It seems that just being involved in a form of worship that connects a person with something larger than the self and provides a notion or experience of transcendence, is life enhancing. Being surrounded by a community of like-minded believers each week, gives the support and nurturance that is of equal importance in later maturity. Organized religion also gives people the continuity of maintaining their own special traditions over the course of a lifetime, or the opportunity to reconnect with the traditions of their childhoods. As we all begin to lose parts of our identities and stature over time, religious identification and community can be vitally important factors in our healthy aging.

However, there is a danger that organized religion can turn into an exclusionist social club: one with the right divinity, the right holy text, and the right beliefs. Sister Joan Chittister, author and Benedictine nun, is very clear in stating that the major error that religion makes, is, "the assumption that having one dimension of it—topic, course, and body of beliefs—we have it all, and if a person does not share this dimension with everyone else, they have no religion at all."[1]

My experience with organized religion is a tale of ambivalence. As a boy, there was no religious presence in our home. My dad occasionally made my sister and me go to the local Catholic Church, but I hated going and eventually that came to an end. A year or so after my mother attempted suicide, my father called us all together and said that he had become a Christian and we were going to go to church as a family. I had never seen my dad so nervous; his hands were shaking and his voice cracking. That Sunday we all appeared at a tiny Baptist Church in the San Fernando Valley. We never really talked in my family, just obeyed what my father said and this was no exception. Eventually, I adapted to going to church on a regular basis and then Sunday school and later a Wednesday night service. I did not know what to think, but I began to enjoy the attention and recognition I received in this congregation. Ours was a start-up church, with some of the members from the sponsoring church and a new Pastor who had been an Associate Pastor before. As time passed I became a youth leader for the church and even preached occasionally.

By the time I was in college, I was an important member of the congregation, and was completely committed to living the life that I felt a Christian was meant to live. In my junior year, the Pastor and his associate called me into their office and told me they thought I was called by God to be a minister, and should start preparing to go to seminary. I was immediately hired as an Associate Pastor to replace my friend and mentor, Reverend Al, as he was leaving to be an Army Chaplain. By that time the church had grown from the small start-up in the back of an orchard, to a fairly substantial middle class Baptist Church, with a congregation of close to a thousand members. I had the responsibility for the junior and senior high groups, and the college group as well.

I got married the summer before I started seminary, and because I was one of the ministers and my then-to-be wife was the daughter of another minister on staff, it was quite an event for the church. Our wedding was one of the highlights of the church year. We went on a honeymoon which proved to be disastrous due to the pressures and expectations on both of us, returned two days early, and tried to get prepared to live on campus in student apartments. I was both scared and elated to break away from my parents and start a life of my own.

Three years of seminary training were transformational for me. Unlike some of the students who just put in their three years and then continued to practice their ministry as they had done previously, I took my education very seriously. So seriously, in fact, that after the adjustment of the first year, I began to question the belief system that had brought me there in the first place. I began to think for myself, to look deeper into the doctrine that I had once accepted on blind faith.

During that first semester, the seminary posted an offer for "sensitivity training" for anyone who was interested. When I read about it, I was filled with anxiety, but knew it was something I had to do. Those who participated were put into two groups for six sessions. Being in a group of my peers to share our feelings brought out many of my deepest fears. Because it was only sensitivity training, we focused more on how we communicated with one another, rather than on deeper emotional issues. After six weeks, the therapist invited me and several others to form a group with the purpose of going deeper into our emotional lives through the process of therapy. I didn't exactly know what this meant, but I knew that I needed to talk about the issues that were causing me so much pain and sorrow. From those initial six weeks, I stayed in therapy, both individually and as part of a group, for the next five years. There was not a session of that therapy that I wasn't filled with anxiety and my stomach in knots, both of which helped me better understand my clients many years later.

Through those turbulent years, everything in my life was a cause for scrutiny. What resulted was not only a transformation emotionally, but a radical shift in my perspective over the last two years of my education. By the time I graduated, I no longer believed in many of the doctrines that were at the heart of orthodox Christianity. Having received a Masters of Divinity with honors, I promptly went to work for United Parcel Service. I left the church to which I had been totally dedicated, and beyond that, I left the community of Christians I had been part of for so many years. Even though I had to start all over again in term of my life goals, I do not regret my decision. I did not fit in the institution that I was being trained to lead, and so choosing another path was the right thing to do.

In rejecting what Sr. Joan Chittister referred to as the major error of religion, believing that a specific dogma holds the "truth," I opened myself to spirituality, that expansive dimension of life through which I am still learning and growing. Spirituality emphasizes internal processes and inner experiences which facilitate the expansion of personal consciousness. It encompasses both a deeper understanding of our own being and a broader connection to other human beings and to the universe at large. Rather than tradition, spirituality seeks new insight into the nature of reality. It is a continual process of self-discovery and self-realization, requiring a person to be tuned into both the conscious and unconscious processes of his or her psyche. But spirituality does not stop at psychological insight; it aims for something more.

We human beings, unlike other sentient creatures, seem to search for a reality above and beyond our own. As we age, we often become, as Loren Eiseley suggests, listeners and searchers for some transcendent realm beyond ourselves.[2] Perhaps it is an inherent need to make sense of existence by putting it in a larger context, one not bound by the limitations of time and space, a context that we do not create, but one in which we find ourselves. To be able to participate in this larger context means transcending ourselves; to overcome, no matter how briefly, the ambiguities and limitations of our existence and make life bearable, and possibly, even wonderful.

The transcendence that makes life more relaxed and enjoyable, includes, in my opinion, more than just believing in that which is wholly other. It implies the ability to get beyond the boundaries of personal ego and invest in that which will live beyond our own existence. Those who can get beyond their own ego identities open themselves to a more encompassing sense of identity by participating in an ongoing creative process through collective values and endeavors. Australian biologist L. Charles Birch, maintains that each of us can find a source of transpersonal meaning by contributing to the completion of a universe which is still in process. "The Universe," he writes, "has always been and is now in the process of being made. It is incomplete. It is lured to further completion."[3] The place where our consciousness meets the "persuasive lure of unrealized possibilities" provides the opportunity for each of us to participate in the creative process of making a more complete world and more ordered lives. To understand this concept, Birch likens persuasive lure to the lure of finding our life purpose. Highly relevant for boomers, finding life purpose is an important yet elusive commodity.

To transcend ourselves is to get a new vision of the meaning of life. Harvard theologian Paul Tillich contended that we could transcend both the heights and depths of existence and participate in something infinite, something eternal. If we are to live zestfully in this stressful world of ours, we need to reach beyond ourselves and transcend the boundaries of our given world, that world which is the total of our beliefs and perceptions about reality.

Later maturity is a perfect time to become aware of the limitations of our myopia and open ourselves to a vision of reality that looks at the whole rather than the parts. It is a good time to re-evaluate the attitudes, values, and notions about reality that we now call our own, and see if they encourage growth or inhibit it. Spirituality calls us to move beyond ourselves, beyond our need to stay secure, stay weak and helpless, and discover our creative potential. In doing so we will begin to see time differently, not as days and months and years that lead in a linear fashion into banality, but as one moment pregnant with possibilities of eternal significance. It may well be that true spirituality is simply being open and accepting of the unexpected, the serendipitous.

Researchers in the field of human aging, however, note the emergence of a tendency toward introversion, or "interiority," as a person travels through later maturity. This includes an increase in contemplation, reflection and self-assessment. Carl Jung affirmed the importance of moving beyond personal facades and societal ideals (persona), to explore the depths of the psyche. This is a movement toward authenticity, a confrontation and discovery of one's personal reality, including both its positive and negative elements. Although seemingly contradictory to the expansion of consciousness in spirituality, interiority is just part of the process of transcendence. In quantum theory, the universe, at the same time, is both within us and all around us. Reaching inward and reaching outward are just different sides of the same coin. Walt Whitman, the great American poet, in his masterwork *Leaves of Grass*, said it this way, "In the faces of men and women I see God, and in my own face in the glass,/ I find letters from God dropt in the street, and every one is sign'd by God's name."

The task for those who desire to live the second half of life with both grace and integrity, is to follow the natural inclination for self-realization without surrendering to isolation or self-aggrandizement. It is to refuse to follow the well-trodden path labeled "aging," but instead to choose the "road not taken" which can lead to an exciting and fulfilling future. It is to disavow the belief that older people are close-minded, set in their ways, and not open to new and potentially mind-expanding experiences.

This, I believe, is the path of spirituality, opening with excitement toward the present and the future rather than remaining in the security of tradition. It means welcoming the growth concepts found in meditation, relaxation techniques, and mind-body awareness. It also encourages an openness to the developments of Humanistic Psychology, such as the use of daily journaling to release insights from the unconscious and the creative use of the arts for the same purpose.

Getting in touch with your spirituality is another reason for daily journaling. I hope by now you are feeling comfortable with your journal and are experiencing more confidence in the material you choose to write about. Research has shown that journaling can not only bring a sense of well-being, but helps strengthen your immune system. Journaling can help us get in touch with our unconscious, bringing out the wisdom of our souls to help us with current issues. In our journaling, we can confront and release anger and resentments, examine our core beliefs, and set forth personal challenges to create new beliefs that actually nurture and support us.

As we continue our journey of years, spirituality may take the form of writing a personal memoir or life review. This can be a creative and fulfilling way to survey and summarize our lives, while at the same time reintegrating past experience and unresolved conflicts. Placing the present in the context of the past allows us to see our lives holistically, bring order to the chaos of experience, acquire new insights and understandings, and develop a more valid, more significant picture of our unique life history.

Part of the zest and vitality in living comes from rediscovering where we have come from, both in terms of the human family and our individual development. That is indeed a second identity formation. The fact is, however, that we never quite arrive. The more we age and change, the more the essential parts of us remain the same. When we write a memoir, we are preserving as well as transforming our identities across time, and gaining a perspective on life that encompasses past, present, and future. We can see where our lives have been and where they are currently, and get a glimpse of where we have yet to go. For me the spiritual path gives us more options than the traditional path. I identify with Robert Frost who wrote these words:

Two roads diverged in a wood, and I--
I took the one less traveled by,
And that has made all the difference
                                        --The Road Not Taken

EXERCISE #9

Writing a personal memoir can be a daunting task. Many of us would like to forget the past and just move on with our lives. The advantages of putting our lives in perspective through the writing of memoirs, I feel, far outweigh the disadvantages. In fact, many universities have classes in the writing of a life review or a personal autobiography, and train counselors in assisting people with this specific task. There are also personal historians who can guide you with both the structure and the process of completing an autobiography.

As you may have noticed, this book has given me the opportunity to share some of my own autobiographical material, and I can personally vouch for the healing that I experienced through the writing.

As I have suggested journaling as a means of getting in touch with repressed memories, unresolved issues, feelings and core beliefs that are hidden from our conscious mind, I am now suggesting that your journal would be a good place to start a personal memoir. Here are a few ideas:

1. Create an outline for your memoir, dividing your life into major time periods, including early childhood, school years, adolescence, early adulthood, later adulthood, and now later maturity.

2. Set down on paper the major events, both positive and negative that happened during those time periods. Write it out as a narrative to the best of your memory. Include the feelings you had then and any feelings you have today about those events. You may want to include information about the house or houses that you lived in to assist your memory.

3. Write about the decisions you made and the actions you took because of the proceeding events. Have those beliefs changed or do they remain the same? Were the actions you took helpful to your life journey or did they make your life difficult? Can you now accept the decisions made and actions taken?

4. What effect did your parents, family and friends have on the course of your life? Are there any unresolved feelings that need to be addressed?

5. The period of adolescence and young adulthood is a good place to write about the relationships you had, having your heart broken, falling in love. What place in your life do these events have? If you got married, write about how you met, your courtship, and the life you had with your partner.

6. Adulthood provides an opportunity to talk about various jobs you had or a career you followed. If you had children, this would be the place to expand on becoming a parent, raising your children, and your relationship with them now.

7. Other events, such as terrific or horrible travel experiences, teachers of memory, how you handled your money, pets that were a significant part of your life, are all things you can include in your memoir.

8. The period of later maturity is your chance to evaluate your life up to date and set out goals that you still wish to accomplish. Are you happy with the way life has gone or are their things that you need help in resolving? If there are things you would like to do over, write them out as a letter to yourself and then say good bye to these fantasies. Unfortunately, you cannot relive the past, only accept that which has happened and let it go.

If you are using your journal, it might be helpful to just write a page each day or the days you are used to writing. It is important to be open to new memories and write about them without judging yourself. Sometimes just writing about things that happened along the way can be healing. If you find yourself being overwhelmed with feelings, anxious or sad, I encourage you to talk with a friend or seek professional advice.

For every reader who decides to write a personal memoir, I hope you find it to be an important experience that enriches your life journey.

EXERCISE #9B

Everyone is made up of conflicting impulses and desires; no one is completely consistent or one-dimensional. When inner conflict becomes too intense, we can become immobilized. Or we can act impulsively without fully realizing what is driving our behavior. This exercise is designed to help you get in touch with any two different and seemingly opposite sides of yourself, by using the technique of an inner dialogue. If you find it helpful you can use the same format to examine other polar opposites, such as weakness-strength, helper-helpless, neat-sloppy, selfish-altruistic, accepting-judgmental, open to new experience-shutdown, optimistic-pessimistic, and so on.

As we age, our tendency is to get stuck in our ways and shut down to new experience. You may think you've seen it all, know the way it always turns out. Let's begin by exploring that side of you which is rigid and closed to new insights, jaded about the world, and that which is flexible and open to new insights and experiences. Change requires that you take a different perspective and allow yourself to be open again.

Remember, this is a process of discovery, so keep a note pad handy to jot down the images and ideas, conflicts, and agreements that emerge.

To begin, get in a comfortable position and close your eyes. Try to relax and slow down inside. Now become aware of your breathing and take three deep breaths, slowly inhaling and exhaling. Now, assume the voice of rigidity, the part of yourself that is resistant to change, that feels closed and guarded. Allow this voice to address the voice of flexibility. You might want to start by saying something like "I feel closed to learning something new," or "it scares me to consider new beliefs," or "why should I take a chance?" It might be something more specific like, "I'm afraid to try meditation because it sounds like new age woo woo to me," or "I don't want to go to a movie at night because I always go during the day." Continue, as the voice of rigidity, to address your flexible side, naming all the various ways and situations in which you can be closed off. Notice how you feel physically as you do this. Are your muscles tensed? Is your face tight? Jaw clenched? Or do you feel drained and defeated? Try to be as detailed as you can about how you feel physically and emotionally as you give this voice full reign. Don't censor or argue with this voice. Let it express itself fully.

Now switch roles and become the voice of flexibility replying to rigidity. You might say something like, "I'd like to take a yoga class," or "I'd like to try taking a community class on making pottery," or "I might meet someone I like if I go to that charity event alone." Try to bring up something that you may not have been open to in the past. What do you say as the voice of flexibility and how do you feel as you say it? Pay attention to your physical and emotional feelings. Do you feel more expansive? Freer? Or does fear creep in? How do you feel in this role, and how do you feel about your rigid side? Now tell your rigid side the benefits of being more flexible. What do you gain by being flexible?

Continue the dialogue by becoming rigidity again. What do you reply to your flexible side? How do you feel as you do this? Now tell your flexible side what you gain by being rigid. Are there disadvantages to being rigid? What part does the rigid side play in your life? Maybe being rigid has helped you to keep all your current values. Maybe it has protected you from your fears. Try to be as specific as possible.

Switch again and become the voice of flexibility. Talk about the disadvantages of being flexible— how friends and family may be frightened by your changes, or how it may have caused you to be more insecure. Go into specific detail about the down side of being flexible.

Now continue this dialogue for a while, switching between rigidity and flexibility and replying to each comment. See what you discover as you explore these two opposite sides of yourself. As I suggested in the previous chapter, spirituality can be described as a spirit of openness to the unknown and unexpected, a way of reaching beyond ourselves to find the infinite in the finite. If we remain overly rigid, we may never reach our creative potential.

Now take out a pen and some paper and write down the insights that emerged in this dialogue, including the following:

1. On which side do you feel most comfortable?

2. Is there any way to have more of a balance in your life?

3. Are there things which frighten you about one of the sides?

4. Can you hold onto traditional values, but still be open to new ideas?

5. Are there any changes you wish to make at this point in your life?

The second half of life provides the opportunity to evaluate where we have been and where we want to go from here. This can be frightening to many people. Remember that fear is just a thought, and really does not mean that much about you as a person. If you are open to it, perhaps this can be an exciting exercise.

FINDING MEANING: AGING WITH INTEGRITY

Rather than love, than money, than fame, give me truth.
--Henry David Thoreau, *Walden*

The concept of integrity is difficult to define, for it is a deeply personal and individual matter. Those who feel that they have achieved it, may conceptualize their experience not as having created or invented something, but as having reached a much sought after destination.

Those who have a sense of integrity have found a deep acceptance of themselves and all of their life experiences. The choice for each of us is to move beyond disappointment and regret about particular events and circumstances in our lives, and choose to accept the entirety of our lives as the way they were meant to be. Integrity flows from the acceptance of the fact that each of our lives are our own responsibility, and that all life experiences, in spite of their ambiguity, as well as all parts of our personalities, in spite of their varying qualities, combine to make each one of us who we are.

The writings of Erik H. Erikson, a practicing psychoanalyst, author and researcher in the field of personality development, are extremely important in understanding the concept of integrity. In *Childhood and Society,* he postulates eight stages in human personality development from infancy to old age. Each stage in this process represents a psychosocial crisis for the growing and maturing individual. Human growth and maturation is seen as a process of facing and resolving specific developmental issues and then moving on to the next. Thus, personality development is seen as highly interrelated and continuous throughout the life cycle. It is the last stage, characterized by the dynamic of *integrity versus despair* that provides the context for this chapter. Encompassing virtually the second half of life, this period of time can be defined for the purposes of this book, as the stage of later maturity.

Erikson himself never gives a definition for the word "integrity," but rather makes some descriptive statements that point to its meaning. The word itself comes from "integer," connoting *undivided, wholeness, health* and *integration*. The process of developing integrity is a process of integration, wherein our lives, experiences, and personalities are accepted and consolidated into the whole of our being. It means accepting ourselves completely, not denying those parts we used to keep hidden from ourselves, but saying "this is who I am," without judgment or denial. It is truly being all that we have been and are now, confidently facing the threat of our death without fear or regret. Erikson felt that if we could not find or actualize integrity, the result would be a life ending in despair. We would feel disgust with ourselves and fear death because we would not feel as if we had fully lived.

Every boomer has the opportunity to come into integrity. It requires that we embrace who we are, accept where we have been in our lives, and boldly face what lies ahead. This wisdom grants depth and purpose to our lives, enabling us to maintain the "wholeness of experience" in spite of declining vitality and approaching death. These are the people we all want to be: people who look back upon their lives with happiness and satisfaction. When we achieve a sense of integrity we can admit to mistakes, but also remember the important and positive experiences in our lives, and draw from these experiences to mentor younger generations and share our wisdom with them.

Wisdom, then, becomes one of the primary ways that integrity expresses itself. Wisdom reflects a personal truth that needs no external validation for it comes from within. The wise person looks within for sources of direction and validation. This kind of wisdom gives each of us the ability to accept both our limitations and our mortality. We live each day more mindfully, with an appreciation for even the daily routines of life.

In the end it all comes down to each of us—our attitudes about ourselves, about the world we live in, about the lives we have lived. Aging zestfully means forgiving our mistakes, coming to know and accept ourselves for who we truly are, not who we wanted to be, and not what we accomplished, or did for a living. In the final stage we can let go of the facades and personas, and learn to be loved and accepted, not by doing, but just by being.

Integrity begins with self-acceptance, a commodity that is not so easy to come by. But as we grow and awaken into it, we will realize that we are not perfect and that not everyone will love, appreciate or approve of who or what we are, and that's OK. With this realization we will find that we stop complaining and blaming other people for the things they did to us (or that we perceived they did to us) and grasp the truth that the only thing any of us can really count on is the unexpected. When we accept ourselves, we will stop judging and pointing fingers, begin to accept people as they are, and overlook their shortcomings and human frailties. When we experience the process of integrity formation, we may find a sense of peace and contentment, as well as a newfound confidence that keeps us open to continued growth and self-awareness.

In the process of experiencing and manifesting integrity, we will, hopefully, come to realize that many if not all of the things we believe about ourselves and the world around us are the result of the messages and opinions that have been passed on to us by significant others and powerful institutions. Our integrity lies in sifting through all of the judgments about who we are, how we should behave, and what constitutes right and wrong. Later maturity is the time to make our own agreements, redefining values for ourselves. It is a time to make a distinction between guilt and responsibility, and learn how to set boundaries that make it possible to say no when we want to, and yes when it is right for us.

Living in integrity brings the realization that we deserve to be treated with love, kindness, sensitivity, and respect, and we won't settle for less. Because we respect ourselves, we will treat others with the kindness and respect they deserve as well. We will also be more discerning of those who do not deserve our respect. Above all else, integrity is an ongoing process, developing within us the sense of gratefulness for all that we have and all that we have been given, and a continual reminder to live in a spirit of thankfulness for the simple things in life that we might have taken for granted before.[1]

One poignant example of an artist who demonstrated integrity despite his own struggles is Vincent Van Gogh. I am visualizing in particular the four paintings of irises and roses that were recently on display at New York's Metropolitan Museum of Art. Although deeply impaired by mental illness, Van Gogh's paintings show his mastery and genius.

Painted nearly 125 years ago as he was preparing to leave the asylum in St.-Remy, where he had spent a year recovering from a form of mental illness said to be triggered by epilepsy (most likely an episode of bipolar disorder), Van Gogh completed the art works in just one week, leaving them in the hospital to dry. He imagined them as a "kind of ensemble" which would express the mood of springtime in Provence, France.

The flowers were chosen from the gardens at St.-Remy, the roses being a special variety distinctive to Provence, referred to as the "hundred-petaled rose." For his colors, Van Gogh, who always sought "simplicity in bright color," chose one of the red lake pigments derived from synthetic dye. Though he knew this color might fade over time, he was attracted to its vibrancy and took the risk to be true to his artistic vision and practice.

Unfortunately, the red lake pigments, which were sensitive to light, did indeed fade, turning the violet of the irises to blue, and the roses from pink to white. The notes for the museum's exhibit of these paintings states: "Never has Van Gogh's observation—'paintings fade like flowers'—been more compelling."

Art Critic Roberta Smith, in her review for The New York Times, writes that seeing these paintings together affirms, "Van Gogh's ability to give flowers the presence of portraits." She also notes that it forces you to "Look more slowly and deeply because there is less to look at." The integrity of the artist to be true to the wholeness of his inner vision, and choose the colors that he felt best expressed that vision—in spite of the possible consequences—is what stands the test of time. The irises and the roses are just as beautiful in blue and white as they were in violet and pink. And like flowers and paintings, it is the nature of human existence for things to fade with time—the color in our cheeks, and the strength in our limbs—but the basic self remains. By accepting ourselves and our lives as a whole, an ensemble of times and events, we follow the path that leads to integrity.

If you go on the Internet you can still see, and perhaps be moved by Van Gogh's brilliant brush strokes, and the emotional intensity they express. He wanted to convey to the viewer what he saw when he looked at those flowers through the lens of his unique self, and that vision still comes through. Knowing that Van Gogh committed suicide just a few short months after their completion, I was touched by "Irises and Roses" in ways that I can't explain. Perhaps I was reminded of the pain my mother must have felt in choosing to end her own life, or just feeling the pain of all those people so tortured they just want consciousness to end. The wholeness of my own life experience, in both its joy and pain, is what I am learning, not only to accept, but embrace. Living and growing with both the positive and the negative of life is what gives us integrity.

Perhaps we can all learn to step outside ourselves and become the observer of our lives. Knowing that we made both good and bad choices along the path that was, and still is our lives, we can cease from making judgments or feeling guilty, and just be at peace with the way it has been. The journey that began with such dependence and innocence, has taken us through many twists and turns, good places and bad ones, happy and sad times. As we move through the second half of life we can begin to slow down and smell the roses and admire the irises along the path. We can learn to accept the things that we cannot change and let go of the pain of our past. We can learn to observe our journey from a much larger perspective, that we were just travelers along the way that millions of others have traveled before. As an observer, we can set aside our egos and be curious rather than anxious about how it is going to turn out. And in that final life transition, perhaps we can say with the poet T.S.Elliot (*Little Gidding*): "We shall not cease from exploration, and the end of all our exploring will be to arrive where we started and know the place for the first time."

EXERCISE #10

A VISIT TO YOUR MEMORIAL SERVICE

Aging with integrity is a process to be lived rather than a goal to be sought. With this in mind consider this final exercise.

Allow yourself to think very far into the future and imagine it is the week following your death. All of your family and friends have come together for a final tribute and memorial service. What are the things that you would hope they say about the following five items:

1. The way you lived your life.

2. The quality of your relationships, both with family and friends.

3. Your character.

4. Your accomplishments.

5. Your legacy.

Well, how did you like the service? In your lifetime, did you experience a sense of integrity and was it reflected in the things that people said about you? Are there things that you would like to do now that would make your final transition one of joy and triumph?

There is only one moment in life, and it is now. Living with integrity is making the most of that moment.

NOTES

CHAPTER ONE

1. Callahan, S., & Christiansen, D. (1974). "The Ideal Old Age." *Soundings*, LVII, p. 4.

2. Mayer, A.J. (1977). "The Graying of America." *Newsweek*, p.50.

3. Hammer, B. (2015). "An Entertainment Power Play: What it's Like to Be a 65-year-old Woman in Hollywood." *Fortune*.

CHAPTER TWO

1. Lawler, K. (2015). "A Conversation with Neil deGrasse Tyson." *AARP Bulletin*, p. 6.

2. Kohn, A. (1986). *No Contest*: *The Case Against Competition*, p.8.

3. Kohn (1986), p. 114.

4. Kohn (1986), p. 180

EXERCISE #1

1. Wilber, K. (1981). *No Boundary*, pp. 119-120.

CHAPTER THREE

1. Chapman, E.N. (2005). *Comfort Zones*, p. 167.

2. Gibran, K. (1985). *The Prophet*, p. 18.

CHAPTER FIVE

1. Chopra, D. (2003). *The Spontaneous Fulfillment of Desire*, p. 79.

2. *Centers for Disease Control and Prevention.* (2013), "The State of Aging and Health in America," p.ii.

CHAPTER SIX

1. Richo, D. (2008). *When the Past is Present*, p.8.

2. Lipton, B. (2005). *The Biology of Belief*, p.164.

3. Siegel, D. (2004). *Parenting from the Inside Out*, p.18.

CHAPTER EIGHT

1. Levine, S. (2009). *Fifty is the New Fifty*, pp. 147-148.

2. Schwartz, P. (2013). "Why are baby boomers so divorce-prone?" *CNN Opinion*.

3. Bair, D. (2007). *Calling it Quits: Late-Life Divorce and Starting Over*, pp. 284-285.

4. Real, T. (2015). *PBS: LifePart 2, Episode 1 Boomer-Marriage Transcript*.

CHAPTER NINE

1. Olson, L. (2011). "Forgiveness: Your Life Depends Upon It," *Family Therapy Magazine*, p.29.

2. Spring, J.A. (2011). "How Do We Forgive Someone Who Isn't Sorry or Alive," *Family Therapy Magazine*, pp. 22-23.

3. Reed, R. (2014). "Prisoners of the Past: Colin Firth Stars in The Railway Man," *New York Observer*.

CHAPTER TEN

1. Chittister, J. (2008). *The Gift of Years: Growing Older Gracefully*, p. 101.

2. Eiseley, L. (1964). *The Unexpected Universe*, p.55.

3. Birch, L.C. (1965). *Nature and God*, p.111.

CHAPTER ELEVEN

1. Adapted from *The Awakening*, Anonymous article.

BIBLIOGRAPHY

Bair, D. (2007). *Calling It Quits: Late-Life Divorce and Starting Over*. New York. Random House.

Birch, L.C. (1965). *Nature and God*. Philadelphia. The Westminster Press.

Brown, S.L., & Lin, I.F. (2012). "The Gray Divorce Revolution: Rising Divorce Among Middle-Aged and Older Adults, 1990-2010." *Journal of Gerontology. Series B: Psychological Sciences and Social Sciences*. 67(6): 731-741.

Callahan, S., & Christiansen, D. (1974). "Ideal Old Age." *Soundings*. LVII. 1:1-16.

Centers for Disease Control and Prevention. (2013). "The State of Aging and Health in America." p.ii.

Chapman, E.N., & Haynes, M.E. (2005). *Comfort Zones*. Axio Press.

Chittister, J. (2008). *The Gift of Years: Growing Older Gracefully*. New York. BlueBridge.

Chopra, D. (2003). *The Spontaneous Fulfillment of Desire*. New York. Harmony Books.

Eiseley, L. (1964). *The Unexpected Universe*. New York. Harcourt, Brace & World.

Erikson, E.H. (1950). *Childhood and Society*. New York. Norton.

Gibran, K. (1971). *The Prophet*. New York. Knopf.

Gottman, J.M., & Silver, N. (2012). *What Makes Marriage Last? How to Build Trust and Avoid Betrayal*. New York. Simon & Schuster.

Hammer, B. (2015). "An Entertainment Power Play: What It's Like to be a 65-year-old Woman in Hollywood." *Fortune*. August.

Hill, R.D. (2008). *Seven Strategies for Positive Aging*. New York. W.W. Norton.

Keen, S., & Valley-Fox, A. (1989). *Your Mythic Journey*. New York. Jeremy P. Archer/Penguin.

Kitchens, J.A. (1994). *Talking to Ducks*. New York, Simon & Schuster.

Kohn, A. (1986). *No Contest: The Case Against Competition.* Boston. Houghton Mifflin Company.

Levine, S. B. (2009). *Fifty is the New Fifty*. New York. Penguin Group.

Lipton, B.H. (2005). *The Biology of Belief.* Santa Rosa. Elite Books.

Lin, I.F. & Brown, S.L. (2012). "Unmarried Boomers Confront Old Age: A National Portrait." The *Gerontologist*. Vol. 52, No. 2. 153-165.

Mayer, A. (1977). "The Graying of America." *Newsweek*. (February 20). 50-55.

Olson, L. (2011). "Forgiveness: Your Life Depends Upon It." *Family Therapy Magazine*. (March/April). 29-31.

Real, T. (2007). *The New Rules of Marriage*. New York. Ballantine Books.

Real, T. (2015). *"Transcript: LifePart2, Boomer Marriage."* www.pbs.org. Episode 1.

Reed, R. (2014). "Prisoners of the Past: Colin Firth Stars in The Railway Man." *New York Observer.* (January 19).

Richo, D. (2008). *When the Past is Present.* Boston. Shambhala.

Richmond, L. (2012). *Aging as a Spiritual Practice.* New York, Gotham Books.

Schwartz, P. (2013). "Why are baby boomers so divorce-prone? *CNN Opinion.* (September 12).

Siegel, D., & Hartzell, M. (2003). *Parenting from the Inside Out.* New York. Jeremy P. Tarcher/ Penguin.

Smith, B.K. (1973). *Aging in America.* Boston. Beacon Press.

Spring, J.A. (2011). "How do We Forgive Someone Who Isn't Sorry or Alive." *Family Therapy Magazine.* (March/April). 21-23.

Vaillant, G.E. (2002). *Aging Well*. New York. Hachette Book Group.

Walsh, R. (2011). "Lifestyle and Mental Health." *American Psychologist*. Advance online publication. (January 17). Doi:10.1037/a0021269.

Wilber, K. (1981). *No Boundary*. Boulder. Shambhala.

48446537R00133

Made in the USA
San Bernardino, CA
26 April 2017